How to Live with OBESITY

Denis Craddock M.D., M.R.C.G.P., D.(Obst.)R.C.O.G.

Heinemann Health Books
London

First published 1975
by William Heinemann Medical Books Ltd
23 Bedford Square, London WC1B 3HT

© Denis F. Craddock, 1975

ISBN 0 4333 06663 6

Reproduced and printed by photolithography and
bound in Great Britain at The Pitman Press, Bath

Contents

Preface

O, that this too, too solid flesh would melt.
SHAKESPEARE

How is it that obesity is included among the many chronic and often incurable disorders which are the subject of this series?

The reason is that the results of treatment of obesity are in general so poor that the majority of people with anything more than a minor weight problem have to live with that problem all their lives. All doctors who have followed up their overweight patients over the years have found this to be true.

The size of the problem is shown by the increase in the number of overweight people in countries with a rising standard of living such as the U.S.A. and Great Britain. In the U.S.A., for example, almost two-thirds of men and women over the age of 40 are overweight and about half of these are considerably overweight. In Great Britain the proportion of overweight women is larger than the proportion of overweight men, but the total represents a huge problem.

Twenty-five years ago, when I first began to practice as a family doctor, I became interested in how much my patients weighed, especially if they themselves were concerned about their weight. I have always kept records of those who have had a weight problem and when I moved to my present consulting rooms, seventeen years ago, I was able to organize my records so that I could follow up my patients. Having a list of patients in the British National Health Service, I was able to make a register of those of each sex born during each year and to compare my overweight patients with a control group of people of the same sex and age. The interesting findings from this survey resulted in my writing a book on obesity for doctors and a short booklet for the general public. This book is a logical sequel.

Introduction

Dr. Denis Craddock has done a real service to the "Control of Obesity" in this book. It has given us a thoughtful, unbiased, and scholarly presentation of the subject of obesity in all of its many aspects.

There is a great deal of research being done at the present time on obesity, because of the lack of knowledge about its underlying causes and the difficulties involved in its control. Numerous fad diets have appeared, and continue to appear, and although these may succeed in a temporary loss of weight, they usually fail to control obesity since they do not enable the individual to maintain a normal weight following a period of dietary deprivation. The modern approach to obesity is proving to have real merit as it recognizes the great importance of psychological factors, as well as the need for dietary control.

Dr. Craddock uses an interesting historical approach, putting obesity in an historical perspective. He talks briefly about the dangers of obesity and gives a discussion of the factors involved in producing obesity. He then goes on to discuss normal weight and gives a brief, easily readable section on nutrients, to enable the individual to have a general understanding about vitamins, calories, and the control of food intake. His discussion of the use of diets is particularly valuable because he takes up the various types of diets and presents his own sample meals, including a description of many of the most popular reducing diets, together with some of the pitfalls involved in snack and social eating, and alcoholic beverages.

His discussion of the role of exercise places this in its proper perspective as a part of a reducing regime. His discussion of the psychological aspects are presented in the light of what relatives, friends, husbands or wives, parents, and the physician, can do to help the obese individual.

The appendix includes a brief table of the calorie value of some of the most common foods.

All in all, this book can be very helpful in enabling the obese individual to understand and successfully handle his problem.

W.H. Sebrell, Jr., M.D.,
R.R. Williams Professor Emeritus
of Nutrition

History

Doctors have been consulted about the problem of overweight at least since the days of the first well-known physician, Hippocrates, who lived from about 460 to about 377 years before the birth of Christ. He observed that "death is more common in men who are naturally fat than in those who are lean". Galen, who lived from about A.D. 130 to A.D. 205 and wrote many books on medical subjects, had this to say about the problem: "The intention of fat is to sustain the animal's heat by combustion in the same way as oil supplies the flame of a lamp, and when that flame is less powerful it is less required that the fat is laid by as in a treasure house". Recent research has shown that fat indeed is used to a large extent for combustion to provide heat, especially in obese people, and that sugar, starch and other carbohydrates are not by any means the only fuel used by the body as had been thought in the early part of this century.

The taking in of nourishment is probably the first thing a baby really enjoys. In a small baby it is associated with the warmth and comfort of the mother's body. When the baby is old enough to be given nourishment away from breast or bottle, the sight and feel of food also bring pleasure.

Eating and drinking have always played a major part in the life of mankind. In primitive societies and in countries where many people go hungry, a man's wealth and standing in society tends to be measured by the

3

weight of his wife or wives. When food is scarce most people eat all they can get and are only too pleased to be able to prove the adequacy of their food intake by becoming fat. In many parts of Africa, young girls are fattened up for marriage. The store of fat also is considered a useful safeguard against possible food scarcity in the future. In primitive societies food was eaten in its natural state and over the last few thousand years the food has usually included meat, fish, or poultry of some sort.

In poor countries such as India, wealthy people are the only ones who can afford to eat enough to become overweight, so that obesity is rare among ordinary working people. When countries become affluent, however, people who have been used to being hungry enjoy having abundant food for the first time in their lives and obesity results. Obesity has been shown to be extremely common for instance among recent immigrants to the U.S.A. and becomes less common in the second and third generations. This is often related to moving up the social scale, where it becomes more important to appear slim.

During the last ten years or so the activities of many scientists and doctors throughout the world have been directed towards finding out why certain people become overweight easily while others, the "lean and hungry" type, may have great difficulty in putting on weight. One famous American physiologist, Dr. Jean Meyer, has written or collaborated in writing over 300 scientific papers on the subject and during the three months before I wrote these lines, 84 papers were published on the subject in the following countries:

Czechoslovakia, France, Germany, Great Britain, Italy, Poland, Rumania, South Africa, Sweden,

Union of Soviet Socialist Republics and United States of America.

The more important points of general interest arising from all this work will be discussed in the next few chapters.

The Dangers of Obesity

It is quite clear from insurance company statistics that people who are overweight live on average a shorter time than those of normal or lean build, and all life insurance companies accordingly charge higher premiums to those who are appreciably overweight. The greater incidence of mortality is brought about mainly by greatly increased occurrence of hypertension and coronary artery disease in obese individuals over forty, and by an increased occurrence of diabetes. Hypertension usually can be treated quite simply once it has been diagnosed, while coronary artery disease is brought about by a multiplicity of factors of which obesity is only one. Both these conditions run in families and it may well be that tendencies toward hypertension and obesity are inherited together. A much higher proportion of small children who are overweight have a blood pressure which is slightly higher than the usual although not of any significance until they are adult. According to recent studies a combination of three factors seems to be responsible for the increase of coronary heart disease incidence as a result of obesity. Excess weight leads to higher cardiac workload and blood pressure; greater caloric intake and blood pressure cause atherosclerosis; thirdly, a decrease in physical activity, usually associated with obesity, brings about a deficient development in collateral circulation.

Diabetes is perhaps the most important condition associated with obesity about which everyone needs to be concerned, as it almost invariably can be prevented by keeping the weight within reasonable bounds. The complications of diabetes can make life unpleasant as they include poor sight, deficient blood supply to the limbs and damage to the nerves supplying the skin, to mention only the major ones. Except for the less common form of diabetes which occurs usually in young slim people, the so-called "maturity onset" diabetes rarely occurs unless individuals have been overweight for fifteen years or longer, and if diagnosed in the early stages it usually can be brought completely under control by the weight loss resulting from a reduction in the intake of sugar and foods containing it.

Other Risks

Getting out of breath easily with slight exertion is perhaps the commonest symptom that takes a fat person puffing and blowing to his doctor, and relief in this case can be rapid. The loss of merely 10-15 pounds (4-7 kg.) in a few months will make a dramatic difference.

The pain arising from worn out weight bearing joints such as the hip, knee and ankle and from minor foot troubles such as corns and bunions causes many other people to hobble along to their doctors. Here again, rapid relief of pain is the rule once weight is lost and the discipline of dieting soon brings its just reward.

Those whose indigestion is brought on by bending forward or lying down are likely to have a defect in the valve mechanism by which the acid contents of the stomach are prevented from flowing into the lower part of the food pipe (oesophagus). It may be that enlargement of the abdomen by fat helps to cause this defect. Whatever the reason, it is certain that weight loss results in relief of symptoms.

What else happens more often to fat people than to thin? Due to the general slowing down of movements, road traffic accidents and indeed accidents of all kinds are more common in overweight people. Surgical operations are also more dangerous. Not only does the surgeon dig deeper to get at internal organs, but fat impairs the action of the lungs and the heart. Most surgeons advise overweight people to lose weight before they are willing to operate on them for non-urgent conditions. Fat women are also more prone to gallstones and dropping of the womb. Fat people usually feel the heat more than thin people and perspire more freely; this is because heat loss from the skin depends on the total surface area of the skin and fat people have a smaller skin surface for their weight than have thin people.

To women, perhaps the most important of the minor alterations in the bodily workings due to overweight is the effect on menstruation. The monthly loss may be delayed and infrequent and in quite young women there may be complete absence of menstrual loss leading to inability to conceive. Here again the results of losing weight can be dramatically effective. Most women who lose an appreciable amount of weight commence menstruating almost immediately and a proportion of them conceive soon afterwards.

Women who start their pregnancy with a high initial weight run a greater risk of toxemia of pregnancy, hypertension and a number of other health hazards.

The Causes of Obesity

Many people think that obesity is commonly due to a disorder of the glands, but this is just not true. A glandular cause for obesity is exceedingly rare and the average family physician probably will see only one or two during his lifetime. However, if a person suddenly becomes overweight without a change in his diet and without altering the amount of exercise he takes, he certainly should consult his personal physician as he may be one of the rare cases which need investigation.

A few people become overweight as a result of treatment with hydrocortisone or one of its derivatives. These steroid hormones are given most commonly for rheumatoid arthritis or asthma, but occasionally also for long-standing skin disease and certain rare blood disorders and they are thought to produce overweight by means of increasing the appetite.

There are many different reasons for an individual becoming overweight but most can be grouped under four headings:

> Hereditary tendencies
> Too little exercise
> Social pressures
> The need to overeat

Hereditary Tendencies

It is common knowledge that overweight runs in families. Most people who are overweight tend to have one or both parents overweight. If one parent is obese about 40-50 per cent of the children become obese; the proportion rises to 70-80 per cent if both parents are obese. If a parent is not overweight then there is usually someone else in the family with the same tendency, a grandparent, aunt, uncle, brother or sister. About two-thirds of my own overweight patients have one or more brothers or sisters who are overweight. Is this due to an inborn tendency or is it, as some doctors think, because overeating tends to be a habit in some families? Whereas it is true that habits of overeating are passed on from parents to children, there is conclusive evidence that there is a strong inborn tendency with most overweight people.

Studies with identical twins provide convincing evidence of hereditary influences. Identical twins grow when the female egg is fertilized by the male sperm and then divides into two. They therefore have identical genes which are the bearers of the hereditary factors in the body cells. If identical twins àre separated from birth and brought up in different families, one would expect their weights to be similar in spite of the different surroundings and different family influences, and this in fact is the case. Their weights are closer to each other than are those of non-identical twins brought up together. Non-identical twins come from separate eggs and are therefore merely children of the same parents who are born at the same time. Their genes can be very different, it being well known that children in the same family can inherit very differing characteristics. The hereditary influence is therefore shown to be stronger than that of the environment.

Studies with adopted children provide further evidence. It has been shown that adopted children take after their real parents as far as weight is concerned and not after the people who have adopted them.

Most people can recall fat children who are similar in looks and behavior to a fat parent, grandparent, uncle or aunt as well as being overweight. Many individuals who are especially fat in certain parts of their body resemble their parents in this. Fat faces, fat chests, fat abdomens, fat buttocks or fat thighs tend to be handed down in families.

People with an inborn tendency to be overweight are in fact different from other people. Recent research has shown that even in childhood some of those who are overweight cannot break down fatty tissue as easily as others and when it is broken down their bodies cannot burn it up to produce heat as easily. In other words, their bodies work differently from thinner people as far as the use of fat is concerned.

Another important factor is that many overweight people have an inherited liking for food which is greater than that of most lean people. Fat children have been shown to have less food dislikes and generally to enjoy eating more than thin children. A well-known American doctor has said, "It seems to me that hunger in the obese might be so ravaging and voracious that we skinny physicians do not understand it".

It is also true that people with a tendency to put on weight easily are inclined to move less quickly than others even before they put on weight, and this tendency is naturally increased when they are heavier. Some individuals expend only half the amount of energy as others even when they are sitting or standing. They tend to be economical in all their movements. On the other hand, the person who is "a ball of fire," who is restless and always on the go, is rarely overweight.

Even if he is merely dictating to a secretary, he will either sit tensely on the edge of a chair and move his arms about or he will walk around the room. Some people of the same height and weight as the active restless individuals actually need only half the amount of calories in order to maintain their weight. So it really is true that some fat people *are* eating less than their lean counterparts.

Too Little Exercise

Lack of exercise is the sole cause of overweight in some people when they give up active sports and exercise or are promoted to a more time-consuming or sedentary job. Being able to afford a car is the downfall of others who previously had to walk or cycle to work. Due mainly to social habits, food intake does not diminish in proportion to the reduction of the amount of exercise. In fact those who exercise least often eat more than those who do a moderate amount of exercise. As work becomes heavier food intake usually increases in proportion; thus blacksmiths eat a lot more than mechanics and drivers. On the other hand, those who do little or no physical work, such as supervisors and clerks, instead of eating less, usually eat more than mechanics and drivers and of course they become fat.

One has in the past probably underestimated the beneficial effects of increased exercise in reducing weight. It would take about ten hours of walking for a person weighing 160 pounds to lose one pound and it has, therefore, been thought to be hardly worth while to include exercise in a weight reducing program. But even this line of reasoning is unsound when considering a long term. Such an individual who walks for an extra 40 minutes per day, e.g. 20 minutes each way to and from work, may lose an ounce of weight daily. This seems hardly worth the extra effort until one realizes that this amounts to nearly half a pound per week, almost two pounds per month and over 20 pounds per year!

Professor Yudkin and his associates in the Department of Nutrition of the University of London have shown that for people of normal weight exercise has the effect of temporarily increasing the rate at which the body works so that calories are burnt up faster. They proved this by over-feeding thin people and showing that their weight did not increase as expected. Over-weight people have lost the capacity to burn up extra food in this way, but can regain it after losing weight.

The excuse many fat people have for not doing exercise is that it only makes them eat more. It is true up to a point that, for instance, a brisk walk can build up a healthy appetite, but I said a healthy appetite. This sort of appetite is satisfied by a *normal* amount of food.

Social Pressures

Social factors play a big part in determining how common obesity is in different social groups in the countries of the Western world. In both the United States and Great Britain, for instance, obesity is less common among the upper classes who can afford the more expensive foods which help to make dieting easier. The wives of many business and professional men aim to preserve a slim appearance as this can be a positive contribution towards their husband's success.

In countries where hunger is common the social incidence is the reverse of that in affluent communities because success in life for a man is often measured by the girth of his wife or wives. In India, for example, obesity occurs mainly in the rich and middle classes, is uncommon in the lower classes and absent in the poor.

Many people still seem to have the impression that it is "healthy" to put on weight. It is certainly true that a person who is putting on weight is unlikely to be suffering from a serious wasting disease such as tuberculosis and therefore overweight implies a certain amount of reassurance about the absence of disease. But tuberculosis is now almost a disease of the past in societies where obesity is rife, and people living in these societies must seriously consider the many disadvantages of being overweight.

National habits also play a part; people of Italian or Spanish origin for example tend to consume large quantities of cereals and dishes cooked in oil. Czechs, for instance, love their food and their traditions include visiting friends or relations on Sundays when large quantities of food are eaten and it is considered impolite to refuse second or even third helpings. In these and other civilized countries social visiting is certainly the downfall of many individuals who enjoy eating and cannot resist the pressures of hostesses who are proud of their skill as cooks and produce overwhelming amounts of fattening delicacies.

Eating habits are important factors in initiating or maintaining obesity in many cultures. In affluent societies or groups, children are impressed from the very earliest days with the necessity of eating a lot to become big and strong. Babies are often overfed with sugar and cereals in the first year of life. Recent research in the United States and Great Britain has shown that this leads to an increase in the number of fat cells in the body which is probably permanent and may initiate a lifelong weight problem. Eating is of course a pleasant social experience and most social functions include eating and drinking. The long established custom of giving food and drink to guests symbolizes affection. Where social visiting is the rule, hostesses tempt their guests with delicacies having a high sugar and fat content and the guests out of politeness usually eat more than they need to satisfy their hunger. As a general rule most people eat quite a lot of things because they like the taste of them rather than because they feel hungry. Social competition is also very common. The visiting ladies observe with great interest everything the hostess has done so that they in turn can attempt to outdo her efforts when they themselves entertain. A hostess is afraid of the gossip of her friends and her hospitality must therefore be lavish.

Most people in their daily living eat at habitual times rather than when they are hungry. In most technologically advanced countries advertising now plays a large part in maintaining the habit of eating for pleasure rather than to satisfy hunger. Roadside advertisements and the daily press make sure that fattening foods cannot escape our notice. Life is especially hard for the dieting television enthusiast who has to sit through many minutes of tempting food commercials between acts of his favorite play or show and, anyway, many people nowadays have the habit of nibbling biscuits, sweets or nuts or drinking beer or soft drinks while watching.

Social Pressures Affecting Men

Business executives in particular have much in their way of life to initiate or maintain obesity. Many of them are "too busy" during the day to take exercise such as walking and are too tired to exercise at the end of the day. Many of them discuss business matters over meals in restaurants at which lavish hospitality is afforded on their firm's expense accounts. When money is no object, alcohol and the more fattening items of food are usually indulged in freely.

Social Pressures Affecting Women

This is truly "a man's world" inasmuch as women suffer much greater temptations to overeat than do men.

They are usually the ones who have the daily temptations involved in the preparation of food. The products of stove and oven must be sampled, the food remnants left by the children must not be wasted and a meal must often be eaten with the husband as well as with the children.

A mother's life is more subject to minor frustrations and the constant decisions and responsibilities involved in looking after children of all ages. The boredom of daily household chores and sometimes, in addition, the strain of full-time work before the babies arrive and again when all the children are of school age make these women cry out for relief; for many, eating is the obvious method of obtaining solace.

When there are no children in the family or when children have left home and perhaps live far away, it us usually the women who bear the brunt of the emotional strain.

Manliness and virility are commonly associated with leanness, or at least an absence of gross obesity. Femininity on the other hand is associated with roundness and plumpness in most cultures. Mothers are usually expected to become matronly in looks by the time their family is complete.

Above all, however, women are subject to the metabolic changes of pregnancy and, in addition, to the emotional upset arising from a first pregnancy which in a civilized society usually occurs five to ten years after the physiological time of the early teens.

The Need to Overeat

Overeating leading to difficulty in weight control often occurs in people who have suffered from lack of affection at some time in their lives, who are at the moment lacking some of the major satisfactions of life or who are being subjected to severe or unusual stresses and strains. These people eat for similar reasons that others smoke, drink, bite their nails or take tranquilizers. Feelings of inferiority are commonly to be found behind the facade of jollity which many fat people present to the world. Being of a good natured disposition, as many fat people are, can arise partly from a basically passive type of personality and partly from deep-seated feelings of inferiority or insecurity. This type of person easily can be presumed upon and become the traditional doormat. Instead of answering back or refusing unreasonable requests, they tend to take refuge in eating; while if they are shy at social gatherings, they also tend to eat instead of talking to people. People who eat for compensation have great difficulty in controlling the desire to eat and if they manage by a great effort of will to lose most of their fat, it is usually put back within a short time. Over many years there may well be a series of quite considerable swings in their weight, but after ten or 20 years they often remain considerably overweight even after one of their episodes of losing weight.

Children who are overweight are often unhappy. Some of them come from broken homes while others were unwanted by their parents who gave them food as a substitute for the deep love that they could not give. Many very happy children, however, have loving parents who cannot resist their children's desires and give them what they want in the way of candy, ice cream, cake and cookies. These items of food are often used as rewards for good behavior or are refused for punishment.

A few people need to be large in size to make up to some extent for feelings of inferiority. To them a well covered frame may have a certain dignity which they are loathe to give up. Some people, however, who feel unloved or unwanted are made even more unhappy by becoming fat and less pleasant to look at. They then tend to think of themselves as undesirable individuals whom nobody could possibly want to love. Feeling unlovable, the urge to eat becomes even greater and a vicious circle is set in motion. These people need help to break the vicious circle by losing the major part of their overweight. This attitude of mind becomes quite an obsession with some people who are, nevertheless, kind, generous, loving and well liked by those who know them well.

Many people start to put on weight when they give up smoking. The reason is partly that smoking takes away appetite in some people but a more important reason is that smoking tends to relieve nervous tension. On giving up smoking, the tense person must now do something else to make him relax and give him some sort of comfort; eating is one of the obvious things to do. My advice to people who want to give up smoking and are afraid of eating too much is to change from cigarettes to a pipe providing that they don't inhale the smoke. As a general rule pipe smokers do not inhale smoke as do cigarette smokers and this may be the main reason why pipe smoking does not have the same serious ill effects on health as do cigarettes. The tremendous increase in chronic bronchitis, coronary artery disease and cancer of the lung is almost entirely confined to cigarette smokers; the risk of developing these diseases in pipe smokers is little different to that of non-smokers.

How to Know
If You Are Overweight

Most people know very well when they are overweight. They only have to see or pick up thick rolls of fat about their bodies for this to be obvious. Of course, a certain amount of fat beneath the skin is normal, particularly in women. Without this essential layer women's limbs would not have the rounded contours which men admire, but thick rolls of fat which can easily be picked up between finger and thumb tell a different story.

There are a few people who are misled by weight tables into thinking that they are overweight when in fact they are not. Weight tables based merely on averages can be very misleading. For one thing they do not take into account the fact that some people are built on slender lines whereas others are of a stocky build and big boned. These latter people, especially if well muscled, could very easily be above average weight without carrying any unnecessary fat.

Weight tables sometimes show increasing weight with increasing age. This is due to the fact that more people become overweight as they become older, but the *average* weight is not necessarily the best weight. Healthy people living a natural life with plenty of exercise and eating natural foodstuffs maintain the same weight until about the age of 60 when the weight begins to fall. Good weight tables would be expected to take into account the differences in build between individuals and also would give the same weight for adults of all ages. The New York Metropolitan Life Insurance Society based their tables on the weights for each height which give the best prospects of long life and produced a series of tables in 1959 giving the desirable weights for men and women over the age of 25 of small, medium and large frames (see Appendix A). Most doctors interested in the problem of overweight now use these tables.

There is no easy way of measuring a person's frame to decide whether it is small, medium or large, although the breadth of the shoulders matches the body framework pretty accurately and people with small hands and feet usually have small bones and small frames as well. If you are in any doubt about the size of your frame try asking half a dozen friends what they think about it.

You will see from the tables what a tremendous difference there is between the weight for a small frame and the weight for a large frame. For most heights it amounts to 30 pounds. Weight tables usually give the weight for a person clothed in normal indoor clothing and this means that a person's stripped weight will be about five pounds less than this figure for a woman and about seven pounds less for a man.

A person's weight varies by up to two or three pounds in a day, usually being higher in the evening. As a pint of water weighs a pound and a quarter, it can be seen that a variation of a pound or more can be dependent on the state of the bowel and bladder. Sweating causing a loss of fluid can also lead to rapid loss of weight which is regained on making up the fluid level by drinking.

If a person is ten per cent above the upper weight limit for his age and build by these tables then it is reasonably certain that he is overweight. Unless he was a fat child or adolescent he will be overweight if he is appreciably above his weight of his early twenties. The fact that he is overweight is confirmed by being able to pick up obvious rolls of fat in certain areas of the body. At the back of the upper arm or on the back below the shoulder blades are two sites where fat always occurs in overweight people. Around the waist, breasts, abdomen, buttocks and thighs are other places where excessive fatty deposits tend to occur. In men fat also can accumulate behind the muscles of the abdominal wall so that these deposits are not accessible to the fingers. However, gradually increasing girth resulting in an inability to zip or button up the trousers shows that fat is likely to have been deposited in this area. If there is any doubt about the matter it is wiser to consult a doctor in case something other than fat is causing the increasing girth. Another condition which should take a person to his doctor is swelling of the ankles or lower legs, particularly if it is of relatively sudden onset as this is likely to be due to fluid rather than fat.

What You Need to Know About Food and How it is Used in the Body

The three main components of foods are proteins, fats and carbohydrates. In addition, certain vitamins and minerals are necessary ingredients of a balanced diet.

Proteins

These are required to build up the body tissues, in particular the muscles, and also to repair them. They do not turn to fat so easily as do carbohydrates. The main protein foods are meat, fish, poultry, eggs, cheese, milk and nuts. There is quite a considerable protein element to be found in peas, beans, lentils, cocoa and most types of cereals including wheat, rye, corn, oats, barley and, to a lesser extent, rice. Strict vegetarians keep well and do not suffer from protein deficiency so that it is not essential for health to eat meat, fish, poultry, eggs, cheese or even milk. However, proteins are very satisfying as foodstuffs, and do not create an artificial appetite as do sweet things.

Fats

These are contained in butter, cream, the fat of meat, fish and poultry and the vegetable oils such as peanut butter, olive, corn, cotton seed and sunflower oil and margarine. Animal fats contain large quantities of the fat-soluble vitamins A and D, and these vitamins are added to margarine. Weight for weight, fats contain more than twice as many calories as do proteins and carbohydrates, but fats satisfy the appetite more completely than other foodstuffs as they remain in the stomach for a longer time.

Fats and Coronary Artery Disease

Coronary artery disease is usually associated with a high level in the blood of a fatty substance called cholesterol. This does not necessarily mean that a high blood cholesterol is the *cause* of the coronary artery disease, but it seems likely that if the level of cholesterol in the blood can be lowered there will be less tendency to develop coronary artery disease. Animal fats give rise to a raised blood cholesterol more readily than vegetable fats and a reduction in animal fats can help to reduce the blood cholesterol level. Vegetable fats which are used, to replace animal fats include corn oil, and margarine with a high polyunsaturated fatty acid content. Polyunsaturated fatty acids are contained in the fat of wild animals but to a much lesser extent in the fat of animals reared for food.

All this concentration on the type of fat eaten is unnecessary in many cases, however, because the level of cholesterol in the blood can often be reduced by cutting out sugar and carbohydrates in the diet.

Carbohydrates

The group of foodstuffs called carbohydrates include the various types of sugar and also the more complex carbohydrates such as starch which form the major part of most cereals and products manufactured from them. Starch is turned into sugar in the body. All carbohydrates are very easily turned into fat in the body.

The Sugars

Natural sugars are found in fruits of all kinds including dried fruits, such as dates, figs, raisins and currants. They also occur to some extent in vegetables such as beetroot, sweet potato, leeks, onions, parsnips, turnips, peas and carrots. Honey, although a natural product, is not a natural food for man as it is provided mainly for bees. Solomon, in his wisdom said, "Keep off much honey". Refined sugar which forms the basis of most of the manufactured foodstuffs in affluent societies is usually made from sugar cane or sugar beet. The brown varieties still have some of the natural flavoring and coloring, but white sugar, which has a much greater world sale, has been so purified that it retains the sweetness of the natural product and nothing more. The worldwide consumption of sugar has increased by five times during the last 100 years. In the United Kingdom the average consumption per head was 14 pounds in 1815 and 120 pounds in 1965.

Somewhat surprising results have been gleaned from worldwide research which has taken place over the last ten years into the fate of foodstuffs in the body. Most refined sugar is called sucrose. One molecule is turned into two molecules of glucose. Now, surprisingly enough, a certain amount of sucrose taken into the body will cause a *rise* in the level of the fatty substance cholesterol in the blood while the same amount of starchy carbohydrates causes a *fall*. Other fatty elements of the blood, notably the triglycerides also are raised by sugar and lowered by complex starchy carbohydrates. Why does this happen? No one knows for certain, but the rapid absorption of sucrose as compared with the slow breakdown of starch to sugar and then its absorption may be a factor. The type of carbohydrate eaten also has an influence on the bacteria living in the bowel and these play a part in the absorption of cholesterol.

The fact that refined sugar has such a different effect in the body from the naturally occurring starchy carbohydrates is one reason why sugar is being increasingly incriminated in the production of several major diseases of civilization, notably coronary artery disease and diabetes. Both these diseases tend to occur about 20 years after a group of people start to eat a civilized diet. A wealth of evidence from all over the world is now accumulating to show that refined sugar, the unnatural food, rather than fat, the natural food, is likely to be the culprit.

One extremely interesting study from Israel compared the Yemenite Jews living in Yemen and those who had been in Israel for 20 years or more. Jews are probably racially the purest of all the races of the western civilized world so that the utmost importance attaches to findings about their dietary habits. The Jews living in the Yemen had a similar dietary intake of animal fat to the Israeli Yemenites and a similar intake of carbohydrates, but they had a lower blood cholesterol level. The only dietetic difference was that the carbohydrate intake of the Yemenite Jews was devoid of sugar and consisted entirely of complex carbohydrates while that of the Israeli Jews contained about 20 per cent of sugar; sugar was presumably responsible for the increased incidence of diabetes and coronary artery disease found among the Israeli Yemenite Jews. A doctor friend of mine practising in the northern Punjab of India deals with the hill people, who are mainly of Tibetan stock, as well as a smaller number of people of the plains who are mainly Indians. Among about 50,000 people, he sees no cases of coronary artery disease and only two or three new cases of diabetes each year. The diabetes occurs among the Indians who come from the south where sweet things are eaten.

The blood cholesterol level can undoubtedly be lowered by reducing or eliminating animal fats from the diet, but these diets usually include a reduction in sugar intake, and a reduced sugar intake on its own without a reduction of animal fats also can cause the blood cholesterol to be lowered. However, it is certainly wise to reduce fats as well as sugars, if a relative has suffered from angina or coronary thrombosis.

Vitamins

As everybody knows, vitamins are essential to health. A person trying to lose weight on a properly balanced diet will get all the major groups of vitamins. Fruit, vegetables, meat, cereals, fish and dairy products are all high in vitamins. The only likely shortage of vitamins while dieting will be for those who are on a low fat diet for a long period of time. Thus, if the total fat intake averages less than one ounce per day over a month or longer, it is wise to take extra fat-soluble vitamins as a precaution. These are vitamins A and D, which can be taken as tablets or in the form of cod liver oil, halibut liver oil or various proprietary preparations. Oily fish such as salmon and tuna also contain vitamins A and D.

Fluids

The amount of fluid drunk during the day is unimportant as far as permanent weight loss is concerned, although weight can certainly be lost rapidly for a short time by a reduction of fluid intake. Boxers can easily "make the weight" by skipping for half an hour and thereby losing fluid from the skin. These weight losses are merely temporary however and once normal fluid intake is resumed the weight goes up again. Permanent weight loss can only be achieved by breaking down the body stores of fat.

In women the amount of water in the body is partially under the control of the female sex hormones, which explains why many women put on several pounds in weight before a menstrual period and lose it when menstruation commences.

Carbohydrates retain fluids. One large carbohydrate meal taken by a person who is trying to lose weight and "goes off the rails" for an hour or two can result in an apparent increase in weight of two or three pounds. This can be very distressing unless it is realized that this weight increase is due mainly to fluid and is therefore only temporary. Dr. Gordon of the University of Wisconsin quotes the case of a man who ate 4,000 calories mainly consisting of carbohydrates on each of two consecutive days. He put on 18 pounds in weight (the amount of fat laid down cannot have been more than two pounds or so) which it took him three weeks to lose!

Salt

Salt intake is unimportant when long term weight loss is being considered. Salt retains fluid so that a reduction of salt intake can result in fluid loss and therefore weight loss. This is only temporary and of no value in the long run.

Minerals

The main essential minerals for health are iron, calcium sodium, potassium and small amounts of magnesium, cobalt, copper, sulphur, fluoride, chlorine and phosphorus. There will be no shortage of any of these ingredients if fruit, vegetables and salads are taken liberally in the diet. Small amounts of iodine are also needed but enough is present in most water supplies and if saltwater fish is taken once a week, iodine supplies are assured.

Changes in Bodily Working (Metabolism) Associated with Obesity

Adaptation to a High Carbohydrate Intake

Carbohydrates tend to be cheap and easy to prepare and at some time or another all overweight people have eaten more carbohydrates than their body has required and the excess has been laid down as fat. Consequently, the body has adapted itself to a high carbohydrate intake by producing an increased output of insulin which the body requires to deal with glucose. (All carbohydrates taken into the body are eventually taken from place to place in the body as glucose.) The extra insulin removes the glucose rapidly from the bloodstream and in some obese people this leads to an almost uncontrollable desire for more carbohydrate to replace it. It can also lead to faint feelings on suddenly changing to a very low carbohydrate diet. These people therefore have an absolute craving for carbohydrates and are in a sense truly addicted to carbohydrates in the same way as a few people whose bodies react in an unusual way to alcohol have a craving for alcohol and become addicted to it. An American physician, Dr. Bloom, has called these people "carboholics" owing to their resemblance to alcoholics and the only real way for them to come to terms with their condition is to abstain completely from carbohydrates in the same way as an alcoholic has to abstain completely from alcohol. This abstention should be permanent. This "addiction" to carbohydrates is uncommon but all obese people tend to have learnt to deal very efficiently with carbohydrates and therefore can easily develop a craving for them.

A Lesser Increase in Metabolism Following Exercise

The carbohydrate tends to be turned to fat rather than to be burnt for energy. It has been shown by Professor Butterfield and his colleagues of Guy's Hospital, London, that glucose is not taken up by the muscles to be burnt in obese people to the extent that it is in the lean. When a substance is "burnt" in the body cells there are of course no flames, but with the aid of oxygen, which is necessary for all burning, the substance disintegrates into other substances and heat is produced. Whereas lean people can "burn off" carbohydrate extra to their needs with the production of heat, obese people have partly lost this capacity. In Professor Yudkin's Department of Nutrition in London, both lean and obese people exercised after a meal of standard size. The increased rate of bodily working, as shown by an increased heat production, was only 28 per cent in obese people, but 56 per cent in the lean. The practical consequence of this increased "thermic effect" in the lean was shown when they deliberately overfed lean young adults and found that they hardly gained any weight at all, whereas when overweight young adults had been overfed at another research center at Edinburgh, they gained weight as expected.

Dealing with Food

Some obese people cannot so easily mobilize fat from their fat stores as can lean people. Adrenalin which normally helps to mobilize fat has been shown by Dr. Gordon of the University of Wisconsin to have a diminished effect in about one-quarter of the obese people he studied. The same has been found to apply to growth hormone which also assists the mobilization of fat from store.

A proportion of obese children show these tendencies to mobilize fat inefficiently, but it has not been decided firmly whether this is a consequence of their obesity or the cause. It is certain that all obese people as a result of their obesity, develop ways of dealing with foodstuffs which are not possessed by lean people. Thus the state of obesity tends to perpetuate itself and most obese individuals can keep a steady overweight by eating the same amount of food as lean individuals who are much less heavy than they are.

Decreased Metabolic Response to Cold

In addition to producing less heat than the lean through less glucose being burnt up in the muscles, obese people do not increase their bodily workings in response to cold in the same way as do lean people owing to the insulating effect of the fat under the skin against the cold. This has been proved experimentally in several different research centers and it is common knowledge that many thin people tend to shiver with the cold. It is this shivering, leading to muscular activity, which helps to burn up glucose so that it is not turned into fat.

This Calorie Business

A calorie is a measure of heat or energy in the same way as a centimeter or an inch are measurements of length. A calorie is the quantity of heat required to raise the temperature of one kilogram of water one degree centigrade. This means that the heat given out by the average human body would be sufficient to boil a small kettle full of cold water every hour!

Fats provide approximately 9 calories per gram.
Proteins provide approximately 4 calories per gram.
Carbohydrates provide 4 calories per gram.

It can be seen that weight for weight fats provide more than twice as many calories as other foods. A man weighing about 70 kilograms (154 pounds) doing a sedentary occupation requires about 3,000 calories per day to provide him with energy. A housewife of average weight needs about 2,500 calories. A man doing heavy work may need as much as 4,000 calories a day or more. The average diet in the Western hemisphere for a housewife might consist of about 70 grams proteins, (280 calories), 70 grams fat (630 calories), 400 grams carbohydrate (1,600 calories).

What Controls the Intake of Food?

Have you ever wondered how it is possible that a person can eat literally tons of food during the course of a lifetime and yet maintain the same weight? It is really rather surprising that this should be so and it is partly due to a tiny part of the brain called the appetite regulating center or appestat. In most people who live a normally active life and have no major stresses or strains affecting them it works as efficiently in keeping their weight at the correct level as does a thermostat in keeping temperature at a certain level. The appestat works well in almost every child who is allowed to eat freely from a wide choice of foodstuffs without being pressed to eat more than he wants and it works well in most adults who stop eating when they feel they have had enough.

What factors affect the appestat?

If the stomach is stretched by anything going into it then hunger is usually relieved and the intake of food ceases. A "meal" of methyl cellulose and water which contains no calories at all often can relieve hunger for an hour or so.

Hunger can be caused by a low level of sugar in the blood and this is one explanation of the fact that in a person who is not a diabetic, injections of insulin, which lower the level of sugar in the blood, can produce a feeling of hunger. In some obese individuals there is a high level of insulin in the blood which removes sugar rapidly from the blood and may make them hungry.

After a meal bodily heat output is increased. This tends to prevent hunger from returning and leads to the spacing of meals.

Dieting to Lose Weight

To lose weight you must take in less food than your body is actually requiring. In this way your body will burn up some of its extra fat to provide energy. If your body needs say 2,500 calories per day and you take in only 2,450 calories per day you are bound to lose weight eventually. Every system of dieting ever produced is therefore designed with the aim of decreasing your calorie consumption below the level you are actually needing at the moment. The diet must therefore be satisfying to keep you from being hungry.

The difficulty is that the overweight person not only needs less calories than the average person, but cannot burn up excess calories in the same way as can lean people. Therefore, in order to lose weight the overweight person may have to eat less than half the amount that other adults in his family or business circles eat. All of us want the easy way out of a difficult situation but **no long term reduction in weight will be achieved without a change in eating habits.**

It should be realized that it will take weeks or months to alter long standing habits of eating but the long-term results will be well worth a sustained initial effort.

How Important Is It to Count Calories?

The answer to this question is that it is not very important at all because the satisfaction value of foods with the same calorific value varies tremendously. In

34

addition, to think largely in terms of calories is to run the risk of becoming obsessional about losing weight and this is neither good for the overweight person nor his relatives. Nevertheless, it is a good plan to have some idea of which foods are very low in calories and can be eaten with impunity and on the other hand which foods are excessively high in calories and should be eaten only under special circumstances, if at all, if weight is to be lost. A list of foods divided into groups by their calorific value is given in Appendix B.

The question of hunger being satisfied is of tremendous importance because it is no good for a person trying to lose weight to starve for much of the day and then to spoil his efforts by being unable to resist eating a huge meal of fattening foods later in the evening when no exercise will follow. Hunger should be satisfied as soon as it commences or not very long after! This means that most people on a diet will need to start off the day with a satisfying breakfast if they are to succeed in losing weight.

Frequency of Eating

Most people lose more weight if they eat three, four or five small meals during the day rather than eating the same amount of food in one or two meals. This is explained by the fact that exercise taken after a meal increases heat loss from the body and therefore increases weight loss. If the metabolic rate is increased in this way four or five times a day more weight loss will occur than if it is increased only once or twice daily. Nevertheless, dieting is an individual affair and some people can lose weight without much difficulty by controlling their appetite during the day and very much enjoying a moderate sized meal in the evening.

For overweight people **sugar is the great enemy.** *Sugar sweetens but does not satisfy.* Some of the facts about sugar will bear reiteration. In people with a tendency to put on excessive weight and who already are eating enough for their needs, sugar turns straight to fat. *The omission of ten heaped teaspoonsful of sugar daily will by itself lead to a loss of one-half pound of fat per week.*

The liking for sweet things (a sweet tooth) must be conquered. This is why the various artificial sweeteners are not really the answer. The appetite for sweet things must be diminished. This may take weeks or months to accomplish, but once accomplished the change is usually permanent. In my own case, I had an extremely sweet tooth until I was in my forties and could not understand how some people were able to finish a meal without eating something sweet. I made several attempts to give up sugar for periods of up to six weeks, but at the end of the time my liking for sweet things had not appreciably diminished. It was not until I determined to conquer the liking for sweet things and persisted in avoiding sugar for a consecutive period of four or five months that I became successful in enjoying drinks and cereals without sugar. Now, several years later, my tastes have altered almost completely. I don't enjoy sweetened drinks or cereals and often prefer to have a second helping of a delicious main dish and miss out the sweet course of a meal altogether.

Once the desire for sugar has been conquered it is not nearly so difficult to resist the temptation to eat sweets, chocolates, biscuits, cakes, jam, honey, syrup, canned fruit, sweetened milk puddings and sweetened fruit drinks. Once the temptation to eat food from the above group has been eliminated the road to permanently successful weight reduction is much smoother. Chocolates, cakes and cookies as well as being delicious are extra fattening as they contain fat as well as carbohydrates.

Carbohydrates Other Than Sugar

Bread, potatoes, rice and other cereals and cereal products are the main forms of high calorie carbohydrates eaten in the West. They all are eventually turned into sugar in the body, but they do not appear to turn to fat as easily as the same amount of sugar. They undoubtedly are less harmful to the person with a tendency to put on weight than is sugar.

Nevertheless, bread, when combined with butter, is so pleasant to eat that many people eat it when they are not hungry, and for this reason it is strictly rationed in most types of diet. Plain breakfast cereals and bran products are usually taken in helpings containing only a small number of calories owing to the bulkiness of the foodstuff as usually marketed. The average helping of breakfast cereals is less than one ounce and provides only about 100 calories. Porridge, rice, macaroni, spaghetti, sago and tapioca take up large quantities of water while being cooked so that an average helping may contain less than 100 calories. Porridge oats in particular takes up about 8 times its own weight of water. Small quantities of all these carbohydrates therefore can be taken by most individuals on a long term diet providing that no sugar is taken with them.

Artificial Sweeteners

It is important to reduce the taste for sweet items of food as well as to avoid eating sugar itself if long term weight control is to be achieved. Nevertheless, there is a place for artificial sweeteners with some fresh fruits, and, in addition, many individuals are unable to tolerate certain types of drinks and food without sweetening agents.

For most purposes and for most individuals ordinary saccharin tablets which contain no calories at all are completely harmless and are as good as anything else. They are also far cheaper than any of the proprietary brands of sweeteners. The following products in tablet or liquid form contain saccharin alone:

Saxin, Sweetex, Bisks, Energen tablets, Hermesetas, Minisax, Supersax, Metasweet and Clickesweet.

Sucron and Sweet 'n Low contain sugar as well as saccharin.

Sorbitol which is used by diabetics contains almost as many calories as sugar and should be avoided.

Fats

Weight for weight fat is higher in calories than any other foodstuff, but to counterbalance this fat satisfies the appetite more completely than any other food. Providing the carbohydrate intake is kept low it is possible that a moderate fat intake may cause weight reduction to occur at a greater rate than if the same number of calories are taken in other forms. When the body is short of carbohydrate and particularly when the carbohydrate intake is below 80 grams (3 ounces) per day, a chemical substance is produced which has the effect of breaking down fat and causing part of the products of breakdown to be lost in the stools and urine. In this way, calories are lost to the body without heat being produced. This substance, discovered in the research laboratories of the Middlesex Hospital, London, by Professor Kekwick and Dr. Pawan and more recently by Canadian workers, has been named Fat Mobilizing Substance. It can be extracted from the urine, purified and utilized for another individual. It has been used experimentally to cause increased weight loss when given by daily injection.

Practical experience has shown that most individuals on a low carbohydrate diet can take all the fat they wish and still lose weight. People are not likely to eat more butter than their body really needs if they don't have much bread to put it on, and it is better to have fresh fruit and cream than to have canned fruit and the syrup which usually goes with it.

Alcoholic Drinks

Alcohol is burnt in the body to provide energy; it releases carbohydrates, and to a lesser extent other foodstuffs, to be turned into fat. Ten pints of beer provide about 2,000 calories, the body's resting requirements for almost a day. It is small wonder therefore that a man who eats his normal meals and then drinks several pints of beer a day puts on weight steadily. A heavy beer drinker usually has to give up drinking or restrict himself to two or three half pints per day to lose weight.

The Free Diet

In my experience most people can lose weight if they want to badly enough by means of one of the so-called free diets in which they can eat as much as they like of certain foods, rationed amounts of a few items of food and nothing at all of a third group of foodstuffs. This type of diet has now been used for over a century.

William Banting, a West End undertaker, published in 1864 his "Letter on Corpulence" giving details of the diet which had been recommended to him by Dr. William Harvey whom he had consulted for deafness. Banting had previously tried all the popular slimming remedies and diets without success, as he was very fond of bread and butter, milk, sugar and pastry. The new successful diet included large amounts of meat and fish, fruit and vegetables and small amounts of wine, but almost completely excluded carbohydrates. Banting was never hungry and yet at the age of 66 managed to lose in a year a total of 46 pounds out of his initial 202 pounds. He lived until he was 82. He wrote, "the great charms and comfort of the system are that its effects are palpable within a week of trial and creates a natural stimulus to persevere for a few weeks more until the facts become established without question". Banting's fame spread so rapidly in Victorian England that his name was soon a household word and to Bant was to slim. More than 50,000 copies of his book eventually were produced. Soon after the last war, Dr. Marriott of the Middlesex Hospital, London, published his well-known diet which was very low in carbohydrates and fats. The Prudent Diet advised by the New York Bureau of Nutrition is based on similar principles. Gordon's diet plan also is similar, but emphasizes the importance of eating six small protein meals daily.

In America, Pennington in 1951 started from the known fact that Eskimos remained lean when their diet consisted mainly of fat meat, but became obese when traders introduced sugar and other carbohydrates into their diet. He helped to popularize a diet of nine ounces of lean meat and three ounces of fat three times a day and advised, in addition, a 30-minute walk before breakfast. This type of diet suited many people in America, and still finds favor there. Donaldson in 1963 in his book, "Strong Meat," advocated an almost identical dietary regime.

Marriott's diet published in 1949 impressed me so much by its common-sense application of sound nutritional principles that I started recommending a diet on similar lines at that time. I felt however that most people could not keep to such a small amount of fat over a long period of time so I modified it by the addition of an ounce of butter or margarine a day and by simplifying some of the details. This modified Marriott's diet has remained my mainstay ever since. Some years ago I collected a series of 79 people who had been on the diet for at least five years. I found that, with the exception of two individuals who had no real intention of keeping to any diet, all of them lost weight although four of them required drugs to help them to keep to the diet. About two-thirds of them lost at least five per cent of their original weight. For example, a person weighing 140 pounds would lose seven pounds or more. One-quarter of them lost over 20 pounds. About half of those who lost an appreciable amount of weight regained much of it by the time the survey ended so that only one-third of the original 79 people had maintained a weight loss of five per cent of their original weight or more by the end of the five-to-eight-year survey period. My results are steadily improving, and after 10 years nearly half of 134 patients had maintained a weight loss.

Rate of Loss of Weight

During the first week many people lose several pounds purely due to the loss of fluid on changing from

a high carbohydrate diet to a low carbohydrate diet.
Add to this the possible loss of two or three pounds of
fat and the total weight loss in the first week can be as
large as 7-10 pounds. A few people who are keeping
strictly to the diet and take a fair amount of exercise
can maintain a weight loss of two or three pounds of
fat for several weeks and therefore a total of 14 or 15
pounds can be lost in the first four weeks. There is no
danger whatever of becoming ill or of feeling weak on
these diets.

John Yudkin, Professor of Nutrition in the University of London, favors a low carbohydrate diet allowing
fat to be taken freely provided the carbohydrate intake
is strictly controlled. He has shown that individuals on
his diet usually take less calories in the form of fat than
they had taken previously! I found this diet a bit too
"free" for some patients and below is set out the
detailed dietary instructions which I now give to almost
all my patients who are commencing a dietary routine.

Low Carbohydrate Reducing Diet

This diet contains no sugar, is low in starch, moderate in fat and high in protein.

(1) Eat and drink as much of the following as you need
to satisfy your hunger:

Lean Meat, including poultry and offal, rabbit, lean
ham and bacon.

Fish

Eggs

Cheese, especially cottage cheese.

Salads

Vegetables

Fresh Fruit (except bananas); or fruit canned without sugar, sweetened with saccharin if necessary. No dried or tinned fruit.

Condiments, sour pickles, thin soups, Worchestershire sauce.

Tea, coffee, low calorie drinks.

(2) You may have:

(a) ½ pint of fresh milk daily (this includes all milk taken in tea, coffee, etc.).

(b) 1 oz. daily of cream, butter, margarine and cooking fat.

(c) Up to 3 ozs. of reducing bread or 6 pieces of crisp bread daily. Wholemeal or brown bread is better for health than white bread. 1 small helping daily of a plain cereal product such as cornflour, macoroni, sago, spaghetti, oatmeal, rice or a non-sweetened breakfast cereal may be taken instead of 1 oz. of bread.

(d) 1 or 2 small potatoes per day.

(3) You may have **nothing else whatever**. Note especially that this means:

No bread, except as above.

No cookies or crackers, cake or pastry.

No cereals, except as above.

No sausages, thick sauces or gravy, puddings, ice cream, peanuts.

No sugar, syrup, chocolate, sweets, cocoa, honey, jam.

No alcoholic drink, sweetened fruit drinks or drinks of unknown content. (See Note 2).

Weigh yourself before you begin, and once a week or once a fortnight afterwards, on the **same scales**, in the **same clothes** and at the **same time of day**.

You should eat three or more meals a day.

You should lose between five and 15 pounds in the first month.

If you cannot keep strictly to your low carbohydrate intake you will need to limit your butter and fats to one ounce per day and cheese to an average of two ounces per day. If you wish to make the diet a little more strict, peas, beans (except string), parsnips, sweet corn, grapes, figs and prunes should be omitted.

Note: (1) Weight can vary up to two or three pounds in the course of a day, usually being higher in the evening.

Note: (2) A glass of beer or wine or a short drink is equivalent in food value to one ounce of bread and may be substituted for it. A drink is best taken with the evening meal.

The Importance of Exercise in Weight Reduction

A person weighing 10 stone who walks three miles each day or cycles for three-quarters of an hour daily, or swims or plays tennis for half an hour daily, will lose *at least* three pounds a month, as well as any weight lost by dieting.

More weight is lost by exercise if it is taken one to two hours after food, as some of the food is turned into heat instead of fat.

Concerning Weighing

Weekly weighing is suggested in the above diet as daily weighing can become an obsession. However, if a person weighs each morning and evening for a week or two it will help him to realize the extent of the daily variations in weight.

The amounts that can be lost by people who adhere strictly to a free diet are based on results obtained with my own patients.

If you are able to keep to a free diet over the years you will be eating a more natural and healthy diet than most people in affluent countries because the modern free diets provide basic vitamins, minerals and body building proteins. It is merely an old wives tale that a person's resistance to infection is lowered by sensible dieting.

Chewing or crunching food is part of the natural un-inhibited pleasure of eating which has been lost by many people who eat modern soft diets, and a good free diet, with emphasis on fresh fruit, vegetables and meat can help to bring back this natural pleasure. It also can help to improve the gums and teeth. The natural friction which the gums get when firm natural foods are eaten helps to prevent the soft flabby gums which are prone to low grade infection (gingivitis), and the absence of refined sugar is a major factor in the prevention of dental decay (dental caries).

Once you have reached your "best weight" you will not lose any more weight even if you keep strictly to the diet. In fact, underweight people can *put on* weight with this type of free diet! Once the desire for sweet things has been conquered and the "best weight" is being approached some people can take certain liberties with the diet without putting on weight again, but a strict watch will always have to be kept on the weight.

A Week of Slimming Meals

The following sample meals for a week do not need to be followed slavishly. They merely serve to give an idea of the satisfying meals containing all the daily requirements of protein, vitamins and minerals, that can be provided on this type of weight-reducing diet. For simplification, the main meal is at midday, but there is no reason why it could not be the evening meal if this is more convenient. Because exercise is beneficial *after* a meal, the heaviest meal should be eaten at midday at least on Saturdays and Sundays.

Note the following points:

(1) Milk must not exceed the daily ration of half a pint.

(2) Bread or toast must be starch-reduced or special formula bread. Starch-reduced crisp breads or rolls can be substituted.

(3) All fruit should be fresh and sweetened as little as possible. No canned or frozen fruits are allowed.

(4) No chocolates, sweets, peanuts or "extras" may be eaten during the day or in the evening. In fact, "no eating between meals" must be a strict rule (but see pp. 72, 73).

(5) If you would like a glass of wine or sherry, or a *single* whisky or gin in the evening, omit the potatoes or bread from the meal.

(6) With average helpings, these sample menus should lead to a *steady* weight loss. If weight loss ceases, cut out or cut down further on potatoes and bread. You will see from the list of foods in Appendix C that vegetables with a relatively high calorific value are peas, broad beans and corn. These should be excluded if weight loss ceases. **Do not cut out meals**.

(7) Weigh yourself once a week on the same scales, at the same time, either naked or in the same clothes. Women may find that they don't lose any weight in the week before their period is due.

Weight-Reducing Diet

DAY 1

Breakfast	Unsweetened fruit juice Scrambled eggs 1 piece of toast with butter Tea or coffee (no sugar)
Mid-morning	Tea or coffee (no sugar)
Midday meal	Vegetable soup Roast chicken Brussel sprouts, small helping buttered carrots, 1 or 2 small potatoes Stewed apple with cream
Afternoon	Tea or coffee (no sugar), lean beef sandwich (1 slice bread and butter)
Evening meal	Slice of melon 3 ozs. cheese, hard-boiled egg Mixed salad (oil and vinegar dressing or lemon juice only) Plain yoghurt without sugar
Nightcap	Milk (left over from daily ration)

DAY 2

Breakfast	Fresh grapefruit Grilled kidneys, bacon and mushrooms 1 piece of toast with butter Tea or coffee (no sugar)
Mid-morning	Tea or coffee (no sugar)
Midday meal	Frankfurters Grilled tomatoes, frozen beans or green salad

	Small helping rice pudding (sweetened with saccharin)
	Grapes (small portion)
Afternoon	Tea or coffee (no sugar)
Evening meal	Chicken or plain omelette
	Spinach
	Fresh fruit
Nightcap	Hot meat or vegetable extract

DAY 3

Breakfast	¾ oz. cornflakes with milk (no sugar)
	Grilled bacon and tomatoes
	Tea or coffee (no sugar)
Mid-morning	Low calorie drink
Midday meal	Tomato juice
	Grilled steak, 1 or 2 small potatoes
	Mushrooms
	Green salad
	1 glass dry white wine
	Egg custard (sweetened with saccharin)
Afternoon	Tea or coffee (no sugar); Cottage cheese and cress sandwich (1 slice of bread and butter)
Evening meal	Smoked haddock
	Frozen peas
	Fresh orange
Nightcap	Hot water and lemon juice

DAY 4

| **Breakfast** | Unsweetened fruit juice |
| | Porridge with salt and milk (no sugar) |

	Grilled kippers Tea or coffee (no sugar)
Mid-morning	Tea or coffee (no sugar)
Midday meal	2 small or 1 large grilled chop Leeks, small helping peas, 1 baked potato Stewed rhubarb with ½ oz. cream or unsweetened evaporated milk
Afternoon	Tea or coffee (no sugar)
Evening meal	Cold meat Mixed salad 1 slice of bread and butter Plain yoghurt without sugar
Nightcap	Milk (left over from ration)

DAY 5

Breakfast	Tomato juice Grilled bacon and poached egg 1 piece of toast with butter
Mid-morning	Unsweetened grapefruit juice with hot water
Midday meal	Beef stew with carrots and onions Stewed gooseberries (sweetened with saccharin) and ½ oz. cream
Afternoon	Tea or coffee (no sugar)
Evening meal	Vegetable soup Fish baked in foil, baked potato and baked tomato Fresh fruit
Nightcap	Hot meat or vegetable extract

DAY 6

Breakfast	Grapefruit Boiled eggs

	1 slice of bread and butter Tea or coffee (no sugar)
Mid-morning	Tea or coffee (no sugar)
Midday meal	Roast lamb with thin gravy Cauliflower (no white sauce), carrots, 1 or 2 small potatoes Fresh fruit salad with ½ oz. cream
Afternoon	Tea or coffee (no sugar)
Evening meal	Liver, bacon and onions 4 ozs. cheese with crisp bread and butter
Nightcap	Lemon juice

DAY 7

Breakfast	Unsweetened fruit juice Scrambled eggs 1 piece of toast with butter Tea or coffee (no sugar)
Mid-morning	Tea or coffee (no sugar)
Midday meal	Steak and kidney pie (small piece of pastry) Cabbage and carrots Stewed pears (sweetened with saccharin) with ½ oz. cream or unsweetened evaporated milk
Afternoon	Tea or coffee (no sugar)
Evening meal	Grilled fish fingers Grilled tomatoes Small helping frozen peas Fresh fruit
Nightcap	Hot grapefruit juice

Other Types of Diet

Counting Carbohydrates

I have frowned on counting calories, but as the free diets are low in carbohydrate some people find that they can keep to them better if they allow themselves only a certain amount of carbohydrate daily and to do this some counting of quantities is inevitable.

Professor John Yudkin first popularized this form of dieting in his book, "This Slimming Business" in 1958. He advised people to take adequate quantities of milk and cheese, meat, fish and eggs, fruit and vegetables and fats, but to ration themselves to 75 grams of carbohydrates daily, reducing this to 50 grams daily if weight loss was too slow. He suggested labeling all foodstuffs with carbohydrate as containing so many units, each unit being equivalent to five grams of carbohydrates. Thus the daily ration of carbohydrates would consist of 15 carbohydrate units (C.U.) reducing to ten C.U. daily if necessary. It could be reduced to five units for really rapid weight loss.

Here is a list of the carbohydrate units contained in the common carbohydrate foods:

Bread, Cakes, etc.

Crisp bread, starch reduced 1
Bread or toast, 1 oz. 3
Reducing bread, 1 oz. 1½
Buns, 2 ozs. 5-8
Cakes and pastries, 2 ozs. 5-8
Roll or scones 5
Starch reduced rolls . . . . ½
Cookies, sweet, 2 small 3

Dumpling 3
Mince pie 4

Fruit and Vegetables

Apples, orange, pear, peach 2
Banana 5
Beans, baked, 2 ozs. 2
Beetroot, small 1
Broad beans, 3 ozs. 3
Cherries, 4 ozs. 4
Corn, 3 ozs. 3
Figs, dried, 2 ozs. 6
Grapes, 4 ozs. 3
Canned fruit in syrup, 4 ozs. 5
Potato, medium size 3

Drinks

Beer, ½ pint 5-8
Sweetened fruit drinks, 1 glass 5
Milk, 1 pint 6
Spirits, 1 tot 4
Sweet wine, 3 ozs. 4
Dry wine, 3 ozs. 3
Stout, ½ pint 7

Cereals, etc.

Breakfast cereal, ½ oz. 3
Porridge, 6 ozs. 3
Macaroni cheese (small portion) 6
Ravioli, spaghetti 10

Sweets, Sugar and Jams

Chocolate, 2 ozs. 5
Ice cream, 2 ozs. 3

Jam, ¾ oz. 3
Sugar, level tsp. 3

Meat Dishes
Frankfurter (large) . . . . ½
Sausage 1½

Puddings
Christmas pudding (small portion) . . . 8
Milk puddings, 4 ozs. 5
Mousse 2
Sago 4
Suet pudding 8
Tapioca 5
Yoghurt (flavored) 4

It will be seen that the C.U. correspond in my diet to Section 2 (the rationed part) which works out at 10-12 C.U. per day and the fruit and vegetable section which can quite easily reach ten C.U. daily or more. The strict carbohydrate counting diet therefore differs mainly from mine by rationing strictly the amount of fruit and vegetables taken.

On this diet it is possible to eat something which is not usually part of my reducing diet such as cakes, ice cream, or sweets without feeling guilty if you ration yourself strictly to the requisite number of C.U. for a 24-hour period. Thus even on a strict diet of only ten C.U. per day by avoiding any bread or fruit you could have a buttered scone and four ounces of chocolate daily. This method of dieting will appeal to some people who cannot avoid eating naughty things occasionally and usually feel tremendously guilty about it. Slimming Magazine Groups have a "Sinners Diet" for this sort of person.

The addition of a moderate amount of fat to a free diet is only successful if a very strict watch is kept on carbohydrates. If a person finds it impossible to keep carbohydrate intake under control then an attempt must be made to ration fats in addition. For example, if you can't keep away from bread don't have too much butter on it, but if you can keep strictly to your bread ration you can put as much butter on your bread as you wish and you will benefit by feeling more satisfied after your meal.

Diets Low in Fat

All low fat diets are very suitable for those who wish to lose weight rapidly and are willing to put up with the unpleasantness of avoiding fat, but few people are able to keep to this sort of routine for more than a few months.

A Free Diet Low in Fat

The Marriott diet was the first of this type to become popular in the 20th century. It is still prescribed by many hospital physicians in Great Britain and copies can be obtained from H.K. Lewis & Co., London, W.C.1.

(1) Eat and drink as much as you like, or can get, of the following:

Lean Meat, including poultry, game, rabbit, hare, liver, kidney, heart, sweetbread—cooked in any way, but without the addition of flour, bread crumbs or thick sauces.

Fish, boiled or steamed only—not fried. No thick sauce.

Eggs, boiled or poached only.

Potatoes, boiled, stewed or baked in skins. Not roast, fried or chips.

Other Vegetables, cooked in any way but without

the addition of fat. Peas and beans should be omitted if weight loss is slow.

Salads and tomatoes without oil or mayonnaise. Beetroots, radishes, watercress, parsley.

Fresh Fruit of any kind including bananas, also fruit canned without sugar. Not tinned or dried fruits (including dates, figs or raisins).

Sour Pickles—not sweet pickles or chutney.

Salt, pepper, mustard, vinegar, Worcestershire sauce (no other sauce).

Saccharin for sweetening. Water, soda water and non-sweetened mineral water.

Tea and Coffee (milk only as allowed below), bouillon.

(2) You may have milk (not condensed) up to half a pint daily.

(3) You may have three very small pieces of bread daily. (Very small means 1 oz. or less.)

(4) You may have **nothing else whatsoever**.

Note particularly that this means:

No butter, margarine, fat or oil (except for cooking meat, but not fish).

No sugar, jam, marmalade, honey, sweets, chocolate, cocoa.

No puddings, ices, dried or tinned fruits, nuts.

No bread (except as above), cake, biscuits, toast, cereals, oatmeal.

No barley, rice, macaroni, spaghetti, semolina, sausage, cheese.

No cocktail savories, alcohol (beer, cider, wines or spirits).

Weigh yourself before you begin and once a week

afterwards, on the same scales, in the same clothes and at the same time of day.

The Prudent Diet

This is used by the New York Anti-Coronary Club to lower serum cholesterol and also to reduce weight if necessary. It is very similar to Marriott's except that at least one ounce daily of vegetable oil or margarine with a high polyunsaturated fatty acid content is allowed. No butter whatever is allowed and only skimmed milk. Calories must be counted.

Meat—beef, mutton, pork: 4 meals/week.
Poultry and veal: 4 or 5 meals/week.
Fish: 4 meals/week.
Eggs: 4 a week.
Fat: at least 1 oz. vegetable oil daily. (This is additional to Dr. Joliff's original Prudent Diet.) Margarine with high polyunsaturated fatty acid content only.
No Butter.
Milk: skim milk only.
Fruit)
Vegetables) ad lib
Grains and Cereal (adequate amounts)
Avoid Ice Cream, hard cheeses, pastry. Take no alcohol or sugar.

For weight reduction limit intake to 1600 calories.

DAILY AMOUNTS FOR WEIGHT REDUCTION

Meat—8 ozs.
Poultry and veal—8 ozs.
Fish—8 ozs.
Eggs—4 *a week*
Fat—1 oz. vegetable oil

Milk—2 cups
Fruit—½ cup citrus fruit, 2 cups other fruit.
Vegetables—3 portions vegetables.
Grains & Cereal—4 one oz. portions.
Cottage cheese—3 ozs.

The diet used by Weight Watchers is based on the Prudent Diet, but goes even further in fat restriction, and limits calories to about 1500 per day.

A Six-meal a Day Diet

Gordon's Diet Plan is a low carbohydrate, moderate fat diet totalling about 1200 calories and including at least six meals a day (my summary).

(1) One egg.

(2) 11 ozs. lean meat:

6 ozs. or more from Group A. Chicken, turkey, pork.
5 ozs. or less from Group B. Fish, lamb, veal, beef.

In Group A. Instead of 1 oz. meat, one tablespoon of peanut butter, twice weekly.

In Group B. 1 oz. cream style cottage cheese, or ½ oz. cheddar, American or Swiss cheese, once a day, or one egg a day.

(3) Seven servings of fat. (1-1/6 ozs.)

One serving:
1 teaspoon corn oil, cotton seed oil or safflower oil.
* 2 teaspoons mayonnaise.
* 1 tablespoon chopped walnuts or 4 half walnuts.
1 teaspoon margarine.

* Not more than two helpings daily.

(4) Two cups skimmed milk.

(5) Two servings fruit.

1 small orange, apple or fig (dried); 1 medium peach; ½ small banana or grapefruit; 2 medium apricots, plums or prunes; 1 cup blackberries, raspberries, strawberries, rhubarb or melon; 10 large cherries; 12 large grapes, 2 dates, ½ cup orange or grapefruit juice; 2 tablespoons raisins.

(6) Two to four cups vegetables. Group A.

Asparagus, cabbage or other greens, celery, chicory, cucumber, egg plant, lettuce, mushrooms, peppers, radishes, string beans, tomatoes, mustard, cress.

(7) One-half slice bread
or
One-half cup vegetables, Group B.

Beets, carrots, onions, peas, turnip, pumpkin.

Suggested Daily Meal Plan

Breakfast	½ cup fruit juice; 1 egg; 1 oz. meat; 1 teaspoon margarine; ½ slice bread; coffee or tea.
Mid-morning	1 cup skimmed milk; 1 oz. meat.
Lunch	3 ozs. meat; vegetable A; 1 teaspoon margarine; 2 teaspoons corn oil; 1 serving fruit; coffee or tea.
Mid-afternoon	2 ozs. meat; ½ cup skimmed milk.
Dinner	3 ozs. meat; vegetable A; 1 teaspoon margarine; 2 teaspoons corn oil; 1 serving fruit; coffee or tea.
Evening	½ cup skimmed milk; 1 oz. meat.

Low Calorie Diets

Those who wish to start weight reduction with a calorie controlled diet can work one out for themselves by weighing their food and calculating the calorie content from Appendix B; but to give them some idea of what a low calorie diet is likely to consist of, here is a sample of a diet containing between 700 and 900 calories daily dependent on the exact size of portions.

800-Calorie Diet

This is likely to contain between 700 and 900 calories. A greater accuracy than this involves weighing of individual items and is only justified for research purposes.

During the day 5 ozs. milk or 10 ozs. low fat milk.

Breakfast   (1) 4 ozs. Tomato juice.
                       or
                One grapefruit,
          (2) One egg boiled or poached
                       or
                1 oz. Oatmeal (before cooking), Shredded Wheat, All-Bran or Weetabix. Milk from ration.
          (3) One cup of black coffee.

Mid-morning Low Calorie Squash or black coffee.

Midday   (1) Half grapefruit
          (2) 2 ozs. lean meat
                       or
                6 ozs. sheep's heart in thin gravy
                       or
                6 ozs. fish baked in foil.
          (3) Mushrooms, runner beans, cabbage, broccoli or sprouts ad lib.

                (4) 1 plain yoghurt
                      or
                   1 apple, orange or pear.

Tea-time   Lemon tea.

Evening meal (1) Clear soup
                     or
                 Half grapefruit.
                (2) 6 ozs. cottage cheese
                     or
                 4 ozs. cold chicken
                     or
                 2 hard-boiled eggs.
                (3) Salad of lettuce, cucumber, grated carrot, celery, radishes and tomatoes.
                (4) 4 ozs. jelly made with gelatine and low calorie squash.
                     or
                 small orange or apple.
                (5) Black coffee.

At night   One glass bouillon or remains of milk.

Note: Unprocessed Bran may be added to a refined cereal such as Corn Flakes or Rice Krispies to a total weight of one ounce.

This diet can lead to a loss of 5-10 pounds in a fortnight if adhered to strictly, but at least 1-3 pounds of this will be due to loss of fluid and will be regained on eating a more normal diet. Some people are happy to carry on counting calories, and most will continue to lose weight on 1,500 calories daily.

Liquid Diets

About ten years ago Metrecal was marketed in the United States and soon after in Great Britain under the name of Metercal. Supplied in fluid form in different flavors or as a powder to which water is added, it provides 900 calories per day in four equal portions with adequate proteins, vitamins and minerals. In both countries most patients managed to survive this sort of diet for three or four weeks at an average weight loss of two or three pounds per week. Complan, the complete food in powder form for invalids, is almost identical to Metercal and approximately half the price. Complan requires flavoring, however.

Some people find that this sort of diet is useful for a quick weight loss, and it can be a pleasant alternative to a strict low calorie diet.

Meal Substitutes

Several biscuits of various makes provide a low carbohydrate low calorie diet. They are intended as meal substitutes or as a complete diet, when they can be used in a similar way to liquid diets. Unfortunately, some of them are sweet and although they are effective for temporary use, they do not help to alter eating habits.

Choosing Your Diet

The diets outlined above offer a wide variety of choice. The straightforward, low carbohydrate free diet is suitable on a long term basis for people who usually eat with others and especially for housewives who find it easier to eat food similar to the rest of the household. It is the safest type of diet for children. Counting carbohydrates is suitable for those people who know that they cannot resist naughty items of food. They can eat certain things without feeling guilty if they cut down on others later in the day. Some people with a very sweet tooth find that they can only do this very gradually, and cannot face cutting out all sweet things immediately. Teenagers will often find this type of diet helpful (see carbohydrate units in Appendix B). To get a flying start with losing weight the 800-calorie diet or liquid diet are suitable, whereas a low carbohydrate, low fat diet is usually best for rapid loss of weight over several months and suits a few individuals indefinitely. For those who have a tendency to peptic ulceration and those who enjoy eating frequently, Gordon's Diet Plan is available. For those on a permanent dietary routine, gimmicky diets can sometimes relieve boredom for a week or two and produce a breakthrough when weight remains stationary.

How Will You Feel While Dieting?

Most people feel perfectly fit while dieting, even if they are doing heavy work, because all these diets are balanced in proteins, minerals and vitamins and body fat is being burnt to produce energy. A labourer under my care lost 25 pounds in five weeks on my free diet and felt perfectly well throughout. Most people feel much fitter when they have lost the first five or ten pounds and some also are relieved of the despair following previous unsuccessful attempts at dieting. Many women gain a lot of pleasure from their new appearance even with a small loss of only five or ten pounds. The only minor upset arising from dieting is that a few people tend to become slightly constipated owing to a less bulky food intake. A few people feel faint with a sudden reduction in the carbohydrate content of the diet (see p. 29). Normal bowel action can usually be restored, however, without the aid of drugs. A few people find that bran flakes or unprocessed bran added to the diet is all that is necessary, while others may require the use of a neutral bulk laxative, like agar agar. These substances absorb water and swell up to add a soft bulkiness to the intestinal contents which allows them to pass along the intestines more normally and causes the normal call to stool to be re-established.

Detailed Notes Concerning Certain Foods

There is a widespread belief that certain foods are not fattening. All foods are fattening—some more than others. The only foods that have hardly any calorie value at all are mushrooms and lettuce.

Bananas: At 22 calories per ounce these are the most fattening of the fresh fruits and unfortunately for the dieter, they are also the simplest and fastest to eat. They should be avoided in dieting households if possible.

Beef: Shin of beef contains just as much protein and just as many vitamins as rump steak.

Brains: At 31 calories per ounce these have less than half the calorie value of most meats.

Bread: Brown bread is no less fattening than white bread. The various starch reduced products have only slightly less starch than ordinary bread and slightly more protein. Nevertheless, they are much lighter than ordinary bread and a *slice* of special bread or a *piece* of crisp bread contains far less calories than a *slice* of ordinary bread.

Calories per slice of bread:

small loaf, medium slice	66
large loaf, medium slice	99
large loaf, thick slice	132

Coca-Cola: This is sweetened, as is Pepsi-Cola.

Coffee: Black coffee only contains a few calories per cup and for those who can learn to enjoy it, is a socially acceptable drink which can take the edge off hunger. Saccharin should be used if necessary to reduce the bitter taste. The popularity of coffee is mainly due to the mild stimulant effect of the caffeine which it contains, and this is the reason why many people who drink coffee late at night find difficulty in sleeping. Those who enjoy the taste of coffee can drink one of the decaffeinated coffees late at night without fear that it will disturb their sleep.

Cornflour: This is mainly carbohydrate in the form of starch. It is less fattening than wheat flour as a thickener for sauces and gravies as it will thicken one-third more liquid than wheat flour.

Crab: About three-quarters of the weight of crab meat is water and most of the rest is protein so that it is a very suitable food for dieters.

Fish: Most types of fish, prepared without the addition of fat, contain about half the calories of most meats. Steamed fish is a little uninteresting, but the taste can be preserved by baking in tinfoil so that none of the juice is lost.

Grapefruit: This is a good fruit for the dieter as it contains even less calories than do oranges. The unsweetened juice is less bitter if diluted with hot or cold water.

Heart: At 27 calories per ounce this is the least fattening of the lean meats.

Honey: Beloved by food faddists, this is almost pure sugar, with minute quantities of vitamins. It is about the only natural foodstuff which can be unwise for dieters to take in any quantity.

Ice Cream: This should be avoided as far as possible as most types contain up to 20 per cent sugar in addition to 11 per cent fat and four per cent protein. The ideal ice cream for the dieter is one made at home from low calorie drinks.

Lemon Juice: The calorific value can be discounted when it is taken diluted for the juice itself contains only eight calories per ounce. Surprisingly, when diluted with hot or cold water, it tastes slightly sweet rather than sour, and is very refreshing. Russian tea is very weak and is served with a slice of lemon, usually in a glass.

Liver: A first class food, rich in protein, iron and vitamin C. It is lower in calorie value than most meats.

Lobster: See Crab.

Milk: Low fat milks afford a saving of about 150 calories per pint as compared with fresh milk. Powdered low fat milk is useful to take away the bitterness of black coffee.

Potatoes: Calorie reduced mashed potatoes with butter flavoring have 17 calories per ounce compared with boiled (23), mashed with milk and butter (27), baked (30, roast (35), and fried (68).

Salad Dressing: Use lemon juice instead, or a low calorie dressing in moderation.

Soup: Clear soups including vegetable soups and bone or vegetable broth are all low in calories, and form a valuable prelude to a meal by taking the edge off the appetite. Beware of most thick soups, especially thick pea soup and noodle soups. Tomato and mushroom soups are the least fattening thick soups.

Tomato Juice: This contains less calories than all fresh

unsweetened fruit juices with the exception of grape-fruit juice.

Tonic Water: This is sweetened with sugar, but unsweetened varieties are now on the market.

Tripe: At 29 calories per ounce this is less than half the calorific value of most types of meat.

Problems For The Dieter

Snacks

Unfortunately the most easily available snacks are usually the most fattening. Biscuits, crackers, bread and butter, cakes and chocolates are rarely absent from the food cupboard. An effort therefore should be made to keep an equally large supply of fruit of all kinds in stock, with the possible exception of bananas. More substantial snacks which are satisfying and easily prepared include cold meat, nuts, cheese, hard-boiled eggs, pickled herring and tomatoes.

Social Eating

Without appearing rude, it is sometimes very difficult to refuse a second helping of a dish which a hostess has spent a lot of time and trouble to prepare. The fattening dishes usually are served towards the end of a meal, however, and the wisest course for the dieter is to have two or three helpings of the early courses avoiding obviously fattening items, by which time it will be hoped that he can refuse a second helping of the sweet course without giving offence.

Packed Meals

Modern vacuum flasks with wide necks can take stews as well as soups, and can even be used to keep solid items such as sausages hot. If you are unable to make use of a knife, fork or plate, the following items of food can easily be eaten with the fingers: hard-boiled eggs; cold leg of chicken; cheese, ham or cold meat wrapped in lettuce leaves; pieces of cold meat or sausage eaten off the skewer on which they were cooked; celery or cucumber filled with soft cheese, potted meat, tuna or salmon.

Drinks

A glass of beer or a small portion of spirits is roughly equivalent to one ounce of bread in calorie value. Bottled beers have slightly more food value than draught beers, and sweet cider, sweet sherry, port or sweet white wine all contain more calories than their "dry" equivalents. Sweet drinks should be avoided both to reduce calorie intake and as part of the general principle of avoiding sweet tasting items of food and drink. Soft drinks, when diluted, contain slightly less calories than beer, and the low calorie squashes which are now on the market contain less than one-tenth the calories of ordinary squashes.

When being entertained, tomato juice is a good substitute for an alcoholic drink, or, with care, one long drink can be made to last the whole evening.

What You Can Do About the Problem

Assess Your Personal Situation Honestly

If you were born with a tendency to be overweight, have always put on weight easily and have considerable difficulty in losing it, there is no getting away from the fact that you have to be careful about the amount and type of food you eat for the rest of your life if you are to avoid excessive obesity. There is at present no easy answer to this problem. Although it is only human nature to seek a "cure" for your condition, only unhappiness can result from attempts to seek an easy way out. It is important for you to be sure in your own mind how serious your weight problem is and how much it affects your life or is likely to affect it in the future before you can make adequate plans to come to terms with it. You might try to answer these questions:

How long have you had a weight problem?

Why have you failed to lose weight in the past; or, if you have lost weight, why have you put it on again?

How much do you enjoy food?

Is it a major interest in your life?

What is your attitude toward exercise?

Do you tend to be slow in your movements?

Do you avoid walking if you possibly can?

Do people in your family circle, at work or among your friends also eat too much of the fattening foods? If so, is it difficult for you to try to avoid eating certain types of food when others

appear to have no worries about eating them?
Do you personally have an emotional need to eat?
Are you unhappy, bored, or tense and do you tend
    to fly to food for comfort?
Do you feel unloved and lonely?
Are you disgusted by the way you look?
Do you wonder how anybody could possibly be-
    come fond of a person disfigured by bulging
    masses of ugly fat?

On the other hand, perhaps you may need to be large in body to bolster up your feelings of inferiority as appears to be the case with some well known personalities. If you are disgusted by the way you look perhaps this may be an expression merely of your own feelings of inferiority. Perhaps other people do not think so badly of you after all. If you are a woman remember that although the modern cult in Western civilization is for women to be slim the majority of men prefer women to look womanly and to differ considerably in figure from themselves. They like a woman to have rounded contours and they like the feeling of comfort that this sort of body can give them physically. Am I trying to persuade you that it is better to be overweight than underweight? No, certainly not. But I am trying to persuade you to accept the best aspects of a situation if it cannot be altered. If as a woman you have a permanent weight problem and are unable to reach your best weight learn to accept a reasonable compromise and settle for being plump, feminine and cuddly.

If you are unhappy, are you really miserable and
    depressed?
Do you sleep badly and wake up early in the
    morning dreading the day ahead?

Do you feel tired in the morning before you have done enough work to earn your feelings of tiredness?

Does life seem hardly worth living?

Have you actually thought at times of putting an end to your miserable existence?

If any of this applies to you then you are not well and can be helped greatly by seeing your own doctor or failing this by consulting a psychiatrist who is known to be sympathetic to ordinary people who feel they cannot cope with life. Even if you are not as depressed as all that, but find that you cannot possibly keep away from food because of the unhappiness and the stresses and strains of your life situation, you can be greatly helped by a sympathetic doctor. But of course there are things you can do yourself if you are bored and frustrated. A man, or a woman for that matter, who does not enjoy his job can give serious consideration to changing it even if this might mean financial loss. A woman who is free from the ties of young children can gain a more interesting life for herself by working part-time or even full-time whether or not she needs the extra money. Even a young housewife with several children below school age can make a positive effort to broaden her horizons by going out of her way to meet people or cultivate some talent. Some young mothers work at home assembling toys or machinery, painting mass produced articles, designing or making knitted or crotcheted garments, making rugs, embroidering or doing typing or secretarial work. Some work at school meal sessions or help with school secretarial work while others spend some evenings working in factories or cafés. Working with food of course is only for the strong-minded. Still others go to evening classes to learn such diverse subjects as art, cookery, hairdressing, foreign languages, guitar playing, country dancing, trampoline or judo.

How Much Do You Really Eat?

Are you being really completely honest with yourself when you consider the amount that you eat? Do you really feel that you "hardly eat a thing"? You may only eat the same amount of food as a person who remains half your weight and this certainly seems unfair, but do you really eat as little as you think? Most of my own patients with difficult weight problems have at some time been asked to write down in detail everything they have eaten for several days. There usually have been some obvious departures from the diets which they said they were keeping and they have often been genuinely surprised to find how many things they have eaten that they should not have. If a person feels guilty about compulsive eating, part of his brain quite genuinely tends to forget some of the times he has eaten the wrong sort of thing or has eaten excessively of anything.

Are you being honest with other people about how much you eat? You will be surprised how much more helpful your doctor, for instance, can be if you are completely honest with him. If you own up to him that you cannot keep strictly to the diet and often have an irresistible urge to eat things you know you ought not, he will respect you more than if you tell him how little you eat and yet manage to avoid losing any weight. He will know in that case that consciously or unconsciously you are deceiving him.

If a person thinks that there is some special reason why they are overweight (and not the real reason that they are eating more than their body needs), then the tendency is to feel that there must be some special way of losing weight other than dieting and the stage is set for a trial of one or the other of the various advertised special ways of slimming, all of which suggest that here is an easy way of losing weight without much effort.

How You Can Keep To a Diet

If you are able to keep to a diet without much difficulty, you have no real problem. Most people with a weight problem know the sort of foods that put on weight, but cannot avoid eating them. You have read in the last chapter about the necessity to satisfy your feelings of hunger. You need to feel full by eating satisfying foods and if these can be of a low calorie nature in addition, so much the better. Once again you must try to find out really what your problem consists of. Do you try to keep to a small amount of food throughout the day and then in the evening find the temptation too great and have a huge meal of fattening food? You are much more likely to lose weight if you have one, two or three substantial meals through the day to stop you from being ravenous in the evening.

Perhaps you are one of those people who cannot avoid nibbling when bored, angry or frustrated. Then for goodness sake keep the very fattening things out of the house if at all possible and replace them with your own favourite protein foods, vegetables and fruits. Why live within constant sight of temptation?

If you love butter, but cannot tolerate margarine or vegetable oil in any form, why not try to persuade the rest of the family to eat one of the very palatable forms of vegetable fat on the market? If sugar is your problem you should spend much time and thought on producing delicious savory dishes, perhaps preceded by an interesting soup or an hors d'oeuvre so that the family has little room for a sweet course. If you are clever enough and persistent enough the rest of the family may come to prefer savoury things to sweet. If biscuits are your downfall, why not forget to replace them while out shopping, or buy some which are not sweet but which still may help to diminish the desire for sweet things in the other members of the family. Tell your family, relatives and friends to stop giving you sweets or chocolates for gifts.

But what else can you do when you have this terrific temptation to have something sweet? People have all sorts of personal answers to this problem. Some chew gum, some chew carrots, some drink large quantities of sweet, low calorie drinks, while some brush their teeth vigorously and enjoy the taste of the toothpaste! Some allow themselves one small bar of chocolate or some other naughty item of food each day which they can enjoy without feeling guilty. It can be made part of a meal or kept in hand for one of those dreadful moments.

Is the preparation of food such a temptation that you cannot avoid tasting everything as you make it? If you can afford to do so why not concentrate on some of the delightful "heat and eat" type meals which are now available in canned and frozen form.

If all else fails, don't be afraid of trying any gimmicky sort of diet which you have garnered from a woman's magazine, a newspaper, or a book, or which has worked for a friend. Most of the diets are quite safe and sensible and will help for a time to relieve the boredom of permanent dieting in a household where other people perhaps can eat well and get away with it. Some of them, however, are by no means nutritionally adequate, so that none should be followed for more than two weeks without medical advice. If by this means or by any other means you can break through a weight barrier, it is possible that you then may be able to maintain your new lower level of weight.

But how else can you help yourself to *keep* to a diet? One way is to catalogue frequently the immense benefit to you of becoming slimmer. Almost every person who slims successfully feels better, looks better and as a consequence gains in self-confidence. This increased self-confidence leads him to be a more complete person who can stand up for himself when necessary, but, on the other hand, is increasingly tolerant of other people's errors and annoying habits.

If by any chance you have lost weight and then put some on again quickly, perhaps while on holiday or at Christmas, then don't let the weight creep up. Go back on a firm diet immediately, once circumstances are back to normal. Remember that part of the weight you have put on so suddenly is fluid and not fat. Things are not really quite so bad as the scales indicate!

Exercise

If you have read and understood Chapter 3 you will realize that exercise can help a great deal in the long term reduction of weight and the maintenance of a lower weight level. *An increased amount of exercise therefore should form part of every weight reducing program.* It is essential, however, especially for people over 40 who have not done any strenuous exercise for some years that the increase in the amount of exercise should be gradual as otherwise a dangerous amount of strain can be thrown on the heart and circulation. Walking, gardening or some other form of non-strenuous exercise should always be indulged in before working up to something more vigorous.

Walking. Three miles a day of walking may well make the difference between being fat and remaining within normal limits. I mention walking first because this is the easiest form of exercise for most people as it involves no expense and can be indulged in almost at will. Even for those whose joints become painful after more than a short distance, frequent limited spells of walking will burn up extra calories.

Walking to and from work can help to save people from the tyranny of the automobile which can enslave its owner to the extent of "needing the car" to go a few hundred yards to post a letter. Walking can also provide a period of respite from the stresses and strains of everyday life and can result in a greater feeling of tranquillity and perhaps a greater appreciation of the simple things of life.

For a person weighing 130 pounds (59 kg.) an extra hour's walking each day, which means approximately three miles at an average pace, would result in a loss of approximately 6.5 pounds (2.9 kg.) in three months, while for a person weighing 225 pounds (102 kg.) the weight loss would be approximately 11.3 pounds (5.1 kg.). It can be seen that extra daily walking is no mean aid to weight loss. To this weight loss must be added an additional "bonus" due to increased heat loss from the temporary increase in metabolic rate resulting from the exercise.

Running. Running can be fun as many thousands of American men are finding out. It is the habit in many

American towns now for men who do not get exercise in their work to run several miles each morning on local athletic tracks such as those belonging to high schools or athletic associations. Providing one is very careful to increase gradually the distance run and takes several weeks to work up to running more than a mile at a time, this can do nothing but good. In some cases there can be the added stimulus of competition or of running against the clock.

Swimming. Swimming is an excellent form of exercise because it can be indulged in by people who have painful knees, hips or ankles which prevent them walking any distance. As is generally known the weight of the body is lessened by the weight of the water which it displaces so that exercise in water throws the least possible amount of strain on these weight bearing joints. A quarter of an hour's actual swimming, as distinct from playing about in the water, uses up as much energy as does one hour's walking. Swimming is also a pleasant form of recreation in which the whole family can take part and if exercise can be fun it is more likely to be taken regularly.

Cycling. Cycling is a dying form of recreation except for the enthusiastic competitor, but it is another very suitable form of exercise for a person who gets pain from the weight bearing joints when walking. In country or surburban areas cycling to work can be an enjoyable alternative to standing in bus queues. For those who live or work near the heavy traffic of towns and cities, a cycling machine to use in the home is an excellent method of keeping fit and losing weight. Leisurely cycling for about three-quarters of an hour is equivalent to about one hour's walking.

Dancing. Dancing is a form of recreation which can

combine an interesting social activity with a useful form of exercise. Shuffling about in the crowded, smoke laden atmosphere of a dance hall is not the most healthy of pursuits, but formation dancing, modern, Latin American or old-time dancing as taught by experts and as practised in small clubs, and evening classes can be graded to suit all types of age and weight.

Golf. The game of golf is suitable for all age groups and is one of the many ways in which walking can be made more interesting. The effect of a person's temperament should be considered however. To some people the frustration of a missed or hooked drive or a bad putt can increase their general irritability and may in fact make them eat or drink more than usual after having played a game!

It need not cost a lot to give the game of golf a trial. Two or three clubs are all that is necessary to start and most areas of the world where golf is played have a few public courses for which there is no membership fee.

Golfers who go on holiday, particularly if they are middle-aged or elderly, are likely to take more exercise than those who do not play.

Physical Training and Gymnastics: This type of exercise forms the basis of the program of many health clubs. Exercising is made interesting, and apart from the more usual equipment, stationary bicycles and rowing machines provide rapid methods of burning up calories. Specific exercises for certain muscle groups can help to make the figure look slimmer; the most important are those to improve the strength of the abdominal muscles and thereby reduce the waist line. You can feel the strain on the two long straight muscles (the recti) which go down the center of the abdomen, whenever an exercise is doing them good. The simplest exercise is to lie down on your back and to sit up slowly without using your hands. Alternatively, in the same position, you can slowly lift up one or both legs while keeping them straight. More complicated exercises include bicycling with legs in the air and press-ups.

Exercise Machines. Beware of static machines, especially the vibratory type in which you are required merely to stand or sit and to allow parts of the machine to vibrate against parts of your body. You will lose more weight if you spend the same amount of time quietly strolling around the gymnasium!

Machines which stimulate muscles electrically so that they contract and are exercised are superior to the vibratory type of machine as they can tone up certain weak muscles to improve the look of your figure. Similar machines employing this method of electrically stimulating muscles have been used for many years in hospital physical medicine departments, but are used less and less as the importance of active exercise is realized. It is possible that electrical stimulation of muscles may lead afterwards to relaxation of tense muscles in areas like the neck.

Clothing

This is a very important subject for women in particular if they are unable to achieve a slender figure. A wise choice of clothing can to a large extent minimize the effect on the eye of ample proportions. A few well chosen dresses of good cut and style are well worth the initial outlay and variations can be achieved by using different accessories.

A few general principles may help in choosing suitable garments. Simplicity should be the keynote, as any sort of fussy clothing such as frills, ruffles, beading, buttons and bows all tend to add bulk. Any tight clothing will tend to emphasize bulges. Colour schemes that blend well are usually better than contrasting ones and dark colours are usually more slimming than light colours.

Large patterns should be avoided. Stripes if worn at all should be vertical rather than horizontal. Two-piece suits, especially of tweedy materials, are usually not flattering and thick-knit (chunky) sweaters and cardigans are not a wise choice. Short skirts in general should be avoided. Straight skirts are more flattering than flared providing they hang well. Trousers in general are best avoided unless they are loose fitting and worn under tunic tops. Stockings and tights should be plain rather than patterned and pale tights should be avoided.

Most fur coats increase the appearance of bulk. Smooth furs are better than rough.

One-piece bathing suits are more flattering than two-piece.

An upswept hair style makes the face look fatter.

A good beautician can advise how to apply brown shaper to slim down cheeks or double chins or to lessen the effects of a broad nose.

If you have a large bust avoid high necklines and elaborate collars. Accessories above the waist should be unobtrusive. Bright colours should be worn only below the waist. Tight belts are unwise.

If you are broad-based, bright and bold accessories of bright colours worn above the waist shift the attention there. Avoid pleated skirts. Sweaters and blouses can be eye-catching.

Notwithstanding all the above suggestions if you really like some article of clothing and it suits you, then wear it!

Foundation Garments. Good and well fitting brassieres and stretch panties or tights can make a tremendous difference to the smartness of a full figure and expert advice is well worth obtaining from experienced corsetieres in the large department stores or from trained representatives who will see you at home. A deep or wired bra can make all the difference to a large bust providing the cup size is correct, the straps are not too tight and there are no rolls of fat pushed under the arms.

Personal Hygiene

Excessive deposits of fat, especially if dependent, cause increased friction and adjoining skin surfaces can easily become chafed and sore. This can even lead to weeping and inflammation when the condition is known medically as intertrigo. The most common places for this to occur are underneath pendulous breasts, below a pendulous abdomen, in the depths of the umbilicus or tummy button, in the groins and where fat thighs rub against each other. A well fitting brassiere of the deep line type or an all in one supporting garment can help to avoid this friction of opposing skin surfaces, but for most women of ample proportions daily bathing and powdering are essential to avoid excessive friction and the formation of unpleasant odors. If "weeping" has occurred a powder with an antifungal ingredient will reduce the prospects of infection of the "thrush" type.

Occupation

It is best to avoid any occupation involving the preparation or serving of food for obvious reasons and a boring job also is likely to lead to an increase in eating.

It is well worth while suffering a loss of income in order to leave a job which increases the temptation to overeat. It is also worth considering changing any job which is frustrating, boring or gives no deep satisfaction for one which involves a vocational interest, especially if to do this means more varied experiences. A man's social standing tends to be correlated with the size of his income, especially in America. But is it not of more value to him in the long run to do work perhaps for less money if that work gives him a feeling of self-respect, makes him happier and more relaxed and less inclined to overeat from boredom or frustration? What is life all about anyway?

An occupation involving walking or any other exercise is obviously preferable to a sedentary occupation and once again the benefit to health can outweigh the disadvantage of a smaller income. Many executive positions in business involve much tension as well as frequent opportunities for eating and drinking too much at business meals.

Group Therapy

Most people find it much easier to alter a deeply ingrained habit if they try to do it together with others. The attempt to break the habit of overeating is no exception. In most western countries group organizations exist to help individuals to lose weight. TOPS in the United States, Weight Watchers in the United States and Great Britain and Slimming Magazine and Silhouette Clubs in Great Britain hold weekly meetings which include a ritual weighing and usually a lecture or discussion. Incentives to keep to a diet include badges or free membership for certain levels of weight loss and in America, the fear of being shown up in public as one of those who has failed to lose weight. Members of groups such as these help each other in the same way as do members of Alcoholics Anonymous by making themselves available on the telephone to give moral support if necessary. Helping to run one of these groups is also a form of voluntary activity which can be of value to the individual concerned.

Apart from the voluntary organizations, public authorities in many countries are now running successful groups. The New York Health Department found that group treatment including close supervision by a physician and nutritionist was more successful than individually supervised weight reduction. Psychologists in Liverpool found that a dietician obtained better results with young mothers taught in a group than when they were given individual instruction. In Great Britain many local authorities have organized groups for the treatment of overweight people, especially children. Some family doctors are realizing that this form of treatment saves them time as well as being helpful to their patients; the detailed running of the group is often left to the practice nurse or health visitor. If your own family doctor does not run such a group, he might be willing to form one if you were willing to do a major part of the organization.

Health Farms or Health Hydros

Most of these places provide a particularly compelling and pleasant form of short term group therapy for those who can afford the fees, which are usually £60-100 per week in Great Britain and $300-1000 in the United States. They are usually situated in pleasant countryside and diversionary activities such as massages, remedial baths, gymnasiums, swimming pools, art therapy, lectures, music and discussions combine to produce a relaxing holiday which reduces the urge to eat. A loss of weight of 10-15 pounds in a fortnight can often result, and although some of this is fluid, more than half the weight loss is likely to be fat.

Unhelpful Measures

Most proprietary slimming remedies are a waste of money. Almost all of them advise a dietary routine as well, and any weight loss is due to the dieting rather than to the particular remedy. The Consumers' Association of Great Britain offered to publish the results if the manufacturers of any of these preparations would carry out scientific trials on their products to prove their efficiency. None of them did so. Slimming remedies in the United States are fully and amusingly exposed in "The Overweight Society," by P. Wyden (1965).

Turkish Baths and sweat corsets help to produce temporary weight loss due to loss of fluid and salt, but no fat is lost and of course the weight is soon put on again.

Spot Reducing

This is not possible to achieve. Fat is laid down in certain places as preordained by hereditary influences, and therefore most fat children put on fat in the same places as their fat parents. On losing weight, fat is lost first from where it has last been put on and eventually if you lose enough weight the fat will disappear from the place which you are worried about. Unfortunately, no amount of massage will "break down fatty globules" and many people have wasted months in applying localized massage to fat thighs and fat midriffs, to their great disappointment. Massage is nevertheless harmless and many people find generalized massage to be relaxing. Some middle-aged or elderly women find to their dismay that they lose fat from their face and neck before it disappears from other parts and losing weight makes them look older although skin wrinkling will improve a little with time. Apart from plastic surgery their problem is unfortunately insoluble.

What You Can Do During Pregnancy

More than half of all pregnant women under my care have tended to put on excessive weight during the early months of pregnancy and I am sure this must apply in every country where there is a high standard of living and the majority of people have all they want to eat. Why is weight put on at this time? One reason is that some women find that eating is the only sure method of relieving the sick feelings of the first three months, while others somehow feel they "ought to eat for two." The main reason however is that during pregnancy there is an increased amount of the hormones of the oestrogen group in the blood stream. Because of this, carbohydrates are more easily laid down as fat and any carbohydrates taken in as food extra to requirements are turned into fat instead of being burnt. Since most women eat more carbohydrates than they need, they will lay down excessive fat.

It is very easy to imagine that increased girth is due solely to the baby and the growth of the womb, and the only way to be sure whether an excessive amount of weight is being put on is to use the scales. What is excessive weight gain in pregnancy? It is generally accepted that a gain in weight of four pounds (1.8 kg.) or more per four-weekly period up to the 20th week and of five pounds (2.3 kg.) or more per four-weeks from then onwards is excessive. Most women can stop their weight gain from becoming excessive or can bring it back to normal again if they drastically reduce their carbohydrate intake by avoiding sugar, sweets, chocolates, cakes, biscuits and crisps and reduce the intake of potatoes, bread and cereals. In fact, about two-thirds of the women to whom I gave this dietary advice during pregnancy responded satisfactorily. Those who did not respond were given a written diet of the free calorie, low carbohydrate type including only one pint of milk per day and, with one or two rare exceptions, they all responded either by gaining less weight in the four-weeks subsequent to the diet or in fact by losing weight. By this means, the average weight gain of those who dieted and showed no signs of toxemia (raised blood pressure and excessive swelling due to fluid) was kept down to a little over 22 pounds (10.0 kg.) as compared with those who had no need for dietary advice and gained a little over 21 pounds (9.6 kg.). The total increase in weight from the ninth week to the 40th week varies with the individual, but as a general rule should not exceed about 28 pounds (13.2 kg.). Some women who are overweight at the beginning of pregnancy manage to keep their weight gain down to as little as ten pounds without any calorie control, which means that they lose upwards of ten pounds or four kilos of fat during the pregnancy and afterwards are able to get into clothes which were unused for several years. If excessive weight is gained during pregnancy, the risk of toxemia, which might injure the baby, is greater and this is another reason for avoiding gaining too much.

What You Can Do If You Are Going Through the Change of Life

First of all don't blame the poor old change of life for your overweight. There is no sudden increase of weight due to the hormone changes which take place at the change of life, or menopause. The proportion of overweight women in an affluent society rises steadily each year from the age of 25 onwards. Pregnancies bring increases in the number of overweight women. Then, as women get into their forties, they usually have less housework to do and most of them undertake less physical work; they have more money to spend and can therefore afford to eat and drink more than they need if they wish to. The result is they take in more calories than they need and gain weight. No, you certainly can't blame the poor old change of life. If anything, with a slight reduction in the amount of the oestrogen group of hormones which helps to lay down fat in pregnancy one would expect fat to be laid down less readily. The menopause merely produces a cessation of the monthly flow and, in some women, hot flushes or hot sweats which can usually be controlled easily by small doses of oestrogens. All the other symptoms put down to the menopause can be accounted for quite simply by the stresses and strains which arise out of changes in a woman's way of life at this time, or changes in her personal relationships with her aging parents, her husband, her growing children, or with people with whom she works.

What You Can Do If You Are an Overweight Diabetic

The overweight diabetic faces a similar problem to any other overweight person, although he has a greater incentive to keep to his diet since the consequences of remaining overweight and losing control of the diabetic condition are so serious. The diabetic is nevertheless subject to the same temptations to overeat and is just as likely to have the same difficulties in keeping to a diet as a non-diabetic.

If he or she is what is known as a "maturity onset" diabetic, i.e. the condition has developed slowly over the age of 40 years after having been overweight for many years and insulin is not needed, then help may be obtained by one of the diabetic tablets which modify the bodily workings in the direction of burning up glucose in the muscles instead of turning it into fat.

What You Can Do If You Suffer From Heart Disease

You have a great incentive to lose weight, as extra weight undoubtedly will lead to some deterioration of your heart condition over the months and years. You should ask your family doctor to help you if you have difficulty in keeping to a diet. You may perhaps be surprised to learn that in your case you can take as much exercise as you like, or can find time for. *Within the limits of your personal tolerance*. This means that you must stop or slow down immediately when you start to get distressed in any way. Pain in the chest, arm or neck coming on with exertion is a warning that exercise must be stopped immediately until the pain passes off. Of course, increasing breathlessness is a sign to stop or slow the exercise. Gentle exercise gradually increasing over a period of days and weeks can in fact be beneficial in many heart conditions. Patients suffering from angina or who have suffered a coronary thrombosis or cardiac infarction at least three months previously have been given steadily increasing amounts of gentle exercise, such as walking or jogging, and have in fact improved the circulation in the coronary arteries which supply the muscle of their heart.

As a general rule, cardiac patients should avoid all strenuous exercises, any sudden exertion, and exercising in very cold weather or immediately after a meal. Any "heart" patient who wishes to increase the amount of exercise he takes should of course consult his family doctor.

What Relations Can Do

An American writer once managed to cut his weight in half, from 350 pounds to 175 pounds. According to him the most trying aspect of this monumental feat was not restricting his food intake, but having to cope with the unhelpful attitude of his friends. A fat person tends to be a figure of fun to many people, a fact which many overweight comedians turn to their own advantage. One reason why some people laugh and look down upon others who are fat arises out of the cruel tendency latent in most of us to build up our own sense of security by acting in a superior manner to those whom we believe to be less fortunate than ourselves. This is the reason why many people look down on minority groups such as Negroes, Jews and unskilled labourers. The same tendency leads some people to sabotage a dieter's efforts because they are afraid that if he loses weight and becomes more self-confident, he will make them feel inferior themselves. This attitude is usually subconscious. For many overweight people, therefore, their relatives and friends actually hinder them in their difficult task.

On the other hand, if relatives are willing to take a helpful and intelligent attitude to an overweight person's problems, they can play a vital role in maintaining his morale and in minimizing the difficulties facing him. If they realize that in most cases an overweight person is not responsible for the fact that he tends by nature to be a rather slow mover, that he cannot help it if he

89

has a tremendous liking for food, and that he has no control over the fact that his body tends to lay down fat easily and give it up from storage with reluctance, it can make a tremendous difference to his whole attitude to life. Praise for success is very necessary for most people who are dealing with a difficult situation and this applies particularly to weight problems. It can be extremely disheartening for a person who has lost say ten to 20 pounds to find that friends or relatives do not even notice any change in his appearance, let alone comment spontaneously on how much slimmer he is looking. This amount of weight loss is obviously noticeable to those who have taken a real interest in a problem so vital to the person concerned. If a relapse has occurred and some weight has been regained, a sympathetic appreciation of his difficulties can help to soften the blow to his self-confidence.

What will help the person with a weight problem most of all, however, is if his relatives make some dietary sacrifice themselves to show that they really mean to help. The adoption of more natural eating habits can do nothing but good for other members of the family. Unfortunately for some dieters, however, not only do some relatives make not the slightest alteration in their own eating habits, but even appear to take a delight in eating obviously fattening foods in the presence of the dieter. Some even look on the whole affair as a huge joke, failing to realize the extent of their cruelty. Tactful relatives will try to eat foods forbidden to the dieter only when they are out of his sight and, when they do eat fattening foods in his presence, will do so discreetly and apologetically. At the table, they will never offer foods which they know should be refused, and will take the same line of action with between meal snacks such as sweets, cakes, chocolates, nuts or biscuits. They will not comment accusingly if food is found to be missing, as the backslider already will be feeling guilty enough about surreptitious eating without it being brought out into the open. The head of the household in particular can play a big part in organizing changes in family habits if his wife or daughter is the one who has to watch her weight.

There are few people these days who take enough regular exercise, and it will encourage an overweight person if other members of the family join him in taking regular active exercise such as walking, swimming and dancing.

Above all, however, relatives can do all in their power to minimize the minor stresses and strains and petty frustrations which help to perpetuate the individual's weight problem. True and genuine affection can help to prevent the excessive eating which partially compensates for an apparent lack of love.

What Husbands Can Do

It should be kept in mind by husbands that women require an outward show of affection much more than do men. The minor courtesies of life matter far more to women than most men realize. Opening doors, helping them on with their outer garments, walking on the outside of the pavement or sidewalk and giving them their rightful place in the family circle when any question of order of importance arises—all are of far more importance to many women than is usually realized. Flowers given either frequently or unexpectedly and cards or surprises on special occasions such as birthdays and anniversaries matter more to most women than cheques and expensive presents.

Some husbands are afraid that if their wives lose weight they will become more attractive to other men, and this shows in their attempts to sabotage the dieting. The husbands are not usually conscious of their motives.

How Parents Can Help Overweight Children

Experience shows that children are not able to keep successfully to a diet unless they themselves have a strong desire to lose weight. It is therefore essential for parents to try to find out why the child has a weight problem and what he or she would like to do about it.

Is there a strong hereditary tendency? This is often the case when children put on weight at a very early age. Has the child been taught bad eating habits from babyhood or infancy? Has he been rewarded by being given chocolates, sweets, ice cream or biscuits for being good or obedient or merely to keep him quiet? Have these things been withheld for punishment? If so, it is hardly surprising that the child should want to have more of these things. Has the child been impressed with the necessity of eating a lot to grow big and strong? Has he often been persuaded to eat more than he really wants to eat? Has he now got into the habit of overeating? Above all, it is of the utmost importance for parents to ask themselves whether it is possible that the child is eating for comfort. Might he feel he is loved a little less than other children in the family? For example, this sometimes can be the case if he was an unwanted addition to the family. Have the parents perhaps tried to make up for their lack of genuine deep love and affection by giving the child the next best thing, which is as much food as he can eat? If a fat child is indeed eating because he is unhappy or feels unloved then it is obviously unkind to add to his unhappiness by trying to deprive him of the feeling of comfort which food brings.

In some fat girls in their early teens a fear of growing up and perhaps of becoming pregnant makes them eat for comfort. They may be rather self-conscious and fearful of any sort of intimate contact with boys and young men.

Whichever of these reasons apply to a particular child, the parents are, after all, responsible for his overweight because they have in fact provided more food than he really needs. Having thought along these lines and having decided that the child does indeed wish to lose weight the kindest thing is to alter the family's eating habits to fit in with his dietary needs. At the same time, it is vitally important to see that he gets his full share of affection and it not made to feel jealous of other children in the family. He will usually not be able to resist accepting chocolates and sweets from his friends, but parents can make sure that he is not given enough pocket money to spend large amounts on buying sweets or ice cream on his way to or from school. Parents should make sure that the same amount of money or more should be spent on fruit, low calorie drinks or special outings to make up for the loss of sweets and biscuits.

The child should be encouraged to join sports clubs or other clubs involving physical activity such as scouts or guides. If he or she is not inclined to join any clubs, some sort of exercise with the family is the best alternative. The importance of the role of exercise in weight reduction is still not generally realized. Many children do not realize how inactive they are compared with others, but that this is true has been shown by taking motion pictures of overweight children playing tennis and comparing them with thin children. Many overweight children do in fact eat only the same amount of food as their friends and in some cases an increase in physical activity is all that is needed to bring them back to being within the normal weight range. Some fat children won't take extra exercise as they may be teased by other children about their looks and slow movements. Where this applies exercise taken with other members of the family is the best answer.

How Parents Can Help Overweight Teenagers

Problems of overweight at this stage of life are often bound up to a large extent with the emotional changes of the teens. Girls are affected more often than boys partly because the changes are often more turbulent in girls and also because girls tend more often to take the passive way out, the way of eating excessively rather than the more active method of adopting an aggressive or destructive attitude.

As most people these days are aware, many of the emotional problems of teenagers arise from the conflict between their desire to become independent individuals coping with life's problems in their own ways and making their own decisions and their child-like need to turn to their parents for protection from decisions and responsibilities which they do not want to take. Parents who appreciate the kind of mixed-up feelings which their teenage children are subject to will endeavour to fulfill a double role in their dealings with them: that of adults treating the young men and women under their care in many ways as equals and allowing them a considerable amount of personal freedom and that of firm foundations to whom the young people can cling whenever they need. This sort of parent will find that their children will need less and less to derive comfort from eating.

Gone are the days when respect was the right of parents. They now have to earn it. They must show by example how to behave as responsible adults and if they are always willing to give time to their children when advice is wanted and if they treat all their children's queries seriously, the children on their side will respond by coming frequently, if indirectly, for advice and will take some note of the advice given even if they do not always heed it!

How Your Doctor Can Help You

A well-known Canadian physician, Professor C. H. Hollenberg of McGill University, has said, "Successful management (of obesity) when it does occur, is the result of a knowledgeable sympathetic physician having the time and the interest to meet repeatedly with a patient who has at least a modicum of insight into the condition and a considerable motivation to reverse it." This is certainly confirmed by my own experience. A doctor who sees his overweight patients regularly and is personally interested in them and their condition will certainly get better results than most. Fortunately, most family doctors like people or obviously they would have preferred to specialize in a branch of medicine where they did not meet people so often. This means that your doctor is on your side from the beginning. If he listens to your troubles, this alone will help you, but you must be completely honest with him. At the initial consultation your doctor may want to check your urine to make sure that you are not developing diabetes. He may also take your blood pressure. If this is high, weight reduction becomes all the more urgent.

I find that most people can keep to a diet for a period of two weeks between the first few appointments. Most successful dieters are then quite happy to be seen monthly. Most National Health Service doctors are unable to see their overweight patients more frequently than this. If an overweight person respects his doctor and wants to co-operate fully with him in carrying out his instructions the doctor's constant encouragement can make the difference between success and failure.

Weight Reducing Tablets

Many people who wish to lose weight ask their doctor for tablets to help them. It is a natural human instinct to want to take the easy way out and it seems so much easier to take tablets to reduce the appetite than to face up to the strict routine of dieting. Nevertheless, as with so many other things in life, the apparently easy way out is not necessarily the best way in the long run, and the only way to lose weight and maintain it at a lower level is to alter eating habits permanently.

Many overweight people fail to realize that weight reducing tablets are *drugs* with capacity to produce unwanted reactions in the body known as "side effects". The side effects can be most unpleasant: nausea, dizziness, headache, palpitations, nervousness, irritability and insomnia are some of them; but, in addition, some of the drugs in current use are members of the amphetamine group. Taking them can lead to increased energy and a feeling of well being, but in some cases, unless strict control is exercised over these weight reducing tablets, a state of drug addiction can result. Once an individual finds that he cannot do without his tablets, he is in a sorry state indeed and his physician may well rue the day he placed him on this type of medication.

The Council of the British Medical Association set up a Working Party to investigate the usefulness of amphetamine preparations. This Working Party recommended in 1968 that "amphetamines and amphetamine-like compounds should be prescribed only for those conditions for which no reasonable alternative exists, . . . more specifically, *"These drugs should be avoided so far as possible in the treatment of obesity,* but if in individual cases the doctor feels they must be used they should be prescribed for a *limited period only."* They also recommended that *"doctors should voluntarily take the same precautions and keep the same records as they already do for those drugs covered by Part I of the Schedule of the Dangerous Drugs Act, 1965."*

Which overweight people are likely to require the help of drugs? In my experience, drugs are useful mainly to help those who have lost a reasonable amount of weight, but have then stuck at a certain weight and have become discouraged. This "weight barrier" can be broken through with the aid of tablets. On the other hand, many doctors find that a modification of diet at this stage is all that is necessary. A wise physician will only allow his patients to continue the use of drugs while they are fulfilling their function and will refuse further supplies when weight loss ceases. He will be especially careful in the supervision of any individual who requires this type of drug for more than three months.

There are other individuals with a constant weight problem who find that they cannot live permanently under conditions where they have to eat differently from the rest of the household in order to prevent themselves from becoming grossly overweight. A short course of tablets for a few weeks once or twice a year can be of tremendous help to these people. There are a very few individuals for whom weight reducing tablets are justified *together with a diet* at the beginning of their attempt to lose weight. People with a tendency to acid indigestion who get pain in the stomach if they don't eat every two or three hours come into this category, as also do a few people who are depressed or tense or a little "backward."

Thyroid or its derivates have been used by some physicians to treat obesity for many years with a varying degree of success. It appears likely that in normal dosage the main benefit was psychological. With the advent of the amphetamines, the use of thyroid declined, but during the last few years physicians in the United States and in Europe have used large doses of thyroid analogues with considerable success in weight reduction. This success in weight reduction has been gained at a price, however, because it has been shown that for these drugs to be really effective they must produce a state of overactivity of the whole body which can lead to illness in some people.

Hormone Injections

Daily injections of chorionic gonadotrophin have been used by a few doctors in the West End of London over the last ten years in conjunction with a 500 calorie diet for a period of about six weeks. Who is going to overeat when they are paying many pounds a week for treatment? It has in fact been shown by a London family doctor that the same weight loss is produced in most people by injections of salt in water! These injections have also been used in the United States and Canada.

Fasting

Your doctor can advise you as to whether an 800 calorie diet is advisable or safe in your particular case. On diets of less than 800 calories body protein may be lost instead of fat. He can advise concerning vitamin supplements and in some cases he may be able to arrange for hospital admission for strict fasting to take place under supervision for longer periods. This facility is available only in a very few hospitals in Great Britain, but is much more readily available in the United States.

Plastic Surgery

In cases of extreme obesity plastic surgery occasionally is advised. The major part of large, pendulous breasts can be removed for comfort and appearance as well as to reduce the total weight by up to ten or 15 pounds (4 to 7 kg.). As much as 50 pounds (over 20 kg.) can be lost by the removal of the huge "apron" of abdominal fat possessed by some individuals, with immediate and tremendous improvement in morale. This fat can of course grow again slowly if a diet is not adhered to subsequently, but localized deposits of fat such as occur on the outer aspects of the thighs in some women do not recur after removal. In some cases plastic surgery can be helpful after weight reduction has occurred if the skin has lost its elasticity and looks baggy and wrinkled.

Bypass Operations

If your bulk is threatening your life and happiness, then your doctor can refer you to a surgeon to consider the possibility of an operation which can direct the food from the stomach into the intestines by a shortened route so as to bypass a large part of the intestines (jejuno-ileal shunt). After this operation there is less time for food to be absorbed so that much of the food taken into the stomach passes through without being absorbed into the bloodstream. This is a major operation. In many of those in whom the operation has been a success diarrhoea persists for many months, and other side-effects may occur. It should only be considered for people who have received no appreciable help from any other treatment and who are in a desperate plight. Most patients who have this operation are compulsive eaters and are double their normal weight.

Psychological Treatment

Any patient who is truly depressed should consult his family doctor for treatment and possible referral to a psychiatrist.

Hypnosis is a method of treatment which can help a few patients after a very careful assessment has been made of their emotional state by a doctor. In a few people hypnosis can help to alter their attitude toward food and feeding so that food is needed as an emotional relief to a lesser extent, but it can never give the wonderful results that some fat people would like to think. There is, in fact, no easy way out and even with hypnosis the individual patient has to cooperate fully in dietary treatment.

Outlook For the Future

For many individuals living in the Western hemisphere where most people eat too much of the wrong food and exercise too little, the pressures of the society in which they live are so great that their obesity is a chronic problem to which they have to try to adjust. The support of an interested family doctor and relatives who understand the difficulties of a person with a tendency to put on weight easily can help to make life tolerable, but if no one around them understands or sympathizes with their predicament, life can indeed be rendered almost unbearable.

Those who are more likely to be able to master their weight problem, to reach their "best" weight and maintain it are more commonly men than women and more commonly married than unmarried. Many of them have a special reason for losing weight either because of a medical condition or because their occupation demands it. A large proportion of them have managed to include an extra amount of exercise in their daily routine.

As far as treatment by doctors is concerned, drugs which modify a person's metabolic processes have only just come into general use. A larger range of these drugs is likely to come on the market in the next few years. "Fat mobilizing substance," a new hormone, has been discovered to be present in the body when there is a deficiency of carbohydrates. This hormone enables fat to be mobilized from storage to be used as fuel. Injections of this substance given to a fat person have been shown to have a similar effect in mobilizing fat to that which occurs naturally in starving individuals. Supplies are still restricted to experimental studies, but in the future it may be possible to market this substance in injectable form or possibly a similar substance to be taken orally. If this becomes a practicable possibility it may have a more dramatic effect than the drugs already in use.

Group therapy holds pride of place in future plans for the rehabilitation of those individuals who have a serious weight problem and most enlightened countries have some form of group therapy for obesity established at least in big cities. Consumer groups or national groups of individuals can help the problem of overweight by promoting drives to reduce the consumption of fattening items such as sugar, sweets and confectionery.

Appendix A
Table of Desirable Weights

Metropolitan Life Insurance Company, 1959
Desirable Weights in Indoor Clothing

Men aged 25 and Over

Height	Weight (pounds)		
	Small frame	Medium frame	Large frame
5' 2"	112-120	118-129	126-141
3"	115-123	121-133	129-144
4"	118-126	124-136	132-148
5"	121-129	127-139	135-152
6"	124-133	130-143	138-156
7"	128-137	134-147	142-161
8"	132-141	138-152	147-166
9"	136-145	142-156	151-174
10"	140-150	146-160	155-169
11"	144-154	150-165	159-179
6' 0"	148-158	154-170	164-184
1"	152-162	156-175	168-189
2"	156-167	162-180	173-194
3"	160-171	167-185	178-199
4"	164-175	172-190	182-204

Table of Desirable Weights

Women aged 25 and Over

Height	Weight (pounds)		
	Small frame	Medium frame	Large frame
4' 10"	92- 98	96-107	104-119
11"	94-101	98-110	106-122
5' 0"	96-104	101-113	109-125
1"	99-107	104-116	112-128
2"	102-110	107-119	115-131
3"	105-113	110-122	118-134
4"	108-116	113-126	121-138
5"	111-119	116-130	125-142
6"	114-123	120-135	129-146
7"	118-127	124-139	133-150
8"	122-131	128-143	137-154
9"	126-135	132-147	141-158
10"	130-140	136-151	145-163
11"	134-144	140-155	149-168
6' 0"	139-148	144-159	153-173

Appendix B

Calorie Values of Common Foodstuffs

Taken from "The Composition of Foods," Medical Research Council's Special Report No. 257 by R. A. McCance and E. W. Widdowson (second impression 1967). All values are for foods as eaten unless otherwise shown. Cooked fruit should be stewed without added sugar, and may be sweetened with saccharine. Each carbohydrate unit is the approximate equivalent of five grams of carbohydrate.

Product	Calories per oz.	Average portion	Calories per portion	Carbo-hydrate units
Fruit				
Apples, fresh	13	one	60	2
Apricots, fresh	8	4 oz.	32	1
Stewed without sugar	6	4 oz.	24	1
canned, sweetened	30	4 oz.	120	5
dried, raw	52	2 oz.	104	5
stewed without sugar	17	4 oz.	68	3
Avocados	25	½ (3 oz.)	75	1

Product	Calories per oz.	Average portion	Calories per portion	Carbo-hydrate units
Bananas	22	1 (4 oz.)	88	5
Blackberries, fresh	8	4 oz.	32	2
Cherries, fresh	11	4 oz.	44	3
Cranberry Sauce	60	1 oz.	60	2½
Black currants (fresh)	8	4 oz.	32	1½
Dates, dried	70	1 oz.	70	4
Figs, dried, stewed without sugar	30	2 oz.	60	3
Fruit cocktail, canned in syrup	27	4 oz.	108	6
Gooseberries, fresh ripe	10	4 oz.	40	2
Grapes, fresh	17	3 oz.	51	3
Grapefruit, fresh (whole fruit)	3	½ (4 oz.)	12	1
Lemon juice	7	½ oz.	3	0
Loganberries, stewed without sugar	4	4 oz.	16	1
Melons	4-7	6 oz.	24-42	2
Olives, green, in brine	24	4 (1 oz.)	24	0
Oranges, fresh	10	1 (6 oz.)	60	3
Orange juice	11	4 oz.	44	2
Peaches, fresh	11	1 (4 oz.)	44	2
canned, sweetened	25	4 oz.	100	4

				2½
Pears, fresh	9	1 (5 oz.)	45	
canned, sweetened	22	4 oz.	88	4
Pineapple, fresh	13	4 oz.	52	2
canned, sweetened	22	4 oz.	88	5
Plums, fresh	10	2 oz.	20	1
canned, sweetened	22	4 oz.	88	4
Prunes, stewed without sugar	19	4 oz.	76	4
Raisins, dried	70	1 oz.	70	4
Raspberries, fresh or stewed without sugar	7	4 oz.	28	4
Rhubarb, fresh raw	2	4 oz.	8	0
Strawberries, fresh	7	4 oz.	28	1.5

Canned fruits are all at least twice the calorie value of their fresh equivalents.

Vegetables

Artichokes, globe, boiled	2	4 oz.	10	0
Jerusalem	5	4 oz.	20	0.5
Asparagus, fresh	5	4 oz. (8 spears)	20	0.5
canned	3	4 oz.	12	0.5
Beans, baked	26	4 oz.	104	4
broad	12	4 oz.	48	3
French or string	2	4 oz.	8	0.5
haricot, boiled	25	4 oz.	100	4
Beetroot, boiled	13	2 oz.	26	1

Product	Calories per oz.	Average portion	Calories per portion	Carbohydrate units
Broccoli, fresh	4	4 oz.	16	0
Brussels sprouts, fresh boiled	5	3 oz.	15	0
Cabbage, fresh boiled or other greens	2	4 oz.	8	0
Carrots, fresh	6	3 oz.	18	1
canned	5	3 oz.	15	1
Cauliflower, fresh boiled	3	4 oz.	12	0.5
Celery, stalk raw	3	3 oz.	9	0
Chicory and endives	3	3 oz.	9	0
Corn, sweet, fresh boiled	24	4 oz.	96	4
Cucumbers, fresh	3	2 oz.	6	0
Leeks, leaves	7	4 oz.	28	1
Lentils, dried	104	1½ oz.	104	3
Lettuce	3	¼ oz.	1	0
Marrow	2	6 oz.	12	0
Mushrooms	2	2 oz.	4	0
Onions, fresh boiled fried	4	4 oz.	16	0.5
	101	2 oz.	202	1
Parsnips, fresh	16	4 oz.	64	2
Peas, fresh	14	4 oz.	56	2
Peppers, green, fresh	7	4 oz.	26	1
Potatoes, chips	68	4 oz.	272	4
boiled	23	4 oz.	92	4

crisps	159	1 oz.	159	1
roast	35	4 oz.	140	4
Pumpkin	4	6 oz.	24	1
Radishes, fresh	4	2 oz.	8	0
Spinach, fresh or canned	7	4 oz.	28	0
Tomatoes, fresh	4	4 oz.	16	0.5
Tomato sauce or ketchup	28	½ oz.	14	0.5
Turnips, boiled	3	3 oz.	9	0.5
Watercress	4	1 oz.	4	0

Nuts

Various, dried	156-189	1 oz.	156-189	1
Chestnuts, fresh	49	2 oz.	96	4

Cereals and their products

Barley	102	1 oz.	102	4
Biscuits, plain	123	2 oz.	226	8
sweet	158	2 oz.	316	7
Bread	65- 72	1 slice	65- 72	3
Breakfast cereals	100-104	1 oz.	100-104	5
Cake, fruit	110-141	2 oz.	220-282	6
sponge	87	2 oz.	174	6
Corn flour	100	1 oz.	100	5
Flour, raw	100	1 oz.	100	4
Macaroni, boiled	32	1 oz.	32	5
Milk puddings, various	36-42	8 oz.	320	8

Product	Calories per oz.	Average portion	Calories per portion	Carbo-hydrate units
Oatmeal, raw	115	1 oz.	115	4
Pastry, shortcrust	132-157	2 oz.	280	3
Rice, polished raw	102	1 oz.	102	4
Suet pudding	105	6 oz.	630	15
Yorkshire pudding	63	4 oz.	252	6
Confectionery				
Chocolate, milk	167	2 oz.	334	5
plain	155	2 oz.	310	5
Honey	82	½ oz.	41	2.5
Ice cream	56	2 oz.	112	3
Water ices	40	2 oz.	80	2
Jams	75	½ oz.	38	2
Low calorie	50	½ oz.	25	1
Jellies, as eaten	23	6 oz.	132	6
Peppermints	111	1 oz.	111	7
Sugar	112	½ oz.	56	3
Sweets, boiled	93	1 oz.	93	4
Toffees	123	2 oz.	246	8
Fats				
Butter	226	¼ oz. (per slice)	55	0

Lard	262	¼ oz.	65	0
Mayonnaise	206	½ oz.	103	0
Peanut butter	170	¼ oz. (per slice)	43	0

Dairy Products

Cheese, Camembert	88	1½ oz.	132	0
Cheddar	120	1½ oz.	180	0
Cottage	30	1½ oz.	45	0
Cream	232	1½ oz.	348	0
Cream, single	62	1 oz.	62	0
double	131	1 oz.	131	0
Eggs, whole	46	1 (2 oz.)	92	0
white	13			0
yolk	100			0
fried	68	1 (2 oz.)	136	0
Milk, pasteurized	19	6 oz. (1 cup)	114	1.5
evaporated	45	1 oz.	41	0.5
condensed, sweetened	100	½ oz.	50	2
dried, skimmed	93	6 oz. (reconstituted)	60	2
Yoghurt, (plain) low fat	15	5 oz.	75	2
with fruit	30-50	5 oz.	150-250	4-6

Meat

Bacon	174	2 oz.	360	0

Product	Calories per oz.	Average portion	Calories per portion	Carbo-hydrate units
Beef, sirloin, roast	109	2 oz.	218	0
hamburger, fried	104	3 oz.	312	0
stewed steak	58	3 oz.	164	0
corned	66	3 oz.	198	0
Brain, boiled	30	3 oz.	90	0
Chicken, boiled or roast (joint)	54	4 oz.	216	0
Duck, roast	89	4 oz.	356	0
Goose, roast	53	4 oz.	212	0
Gravy, thin	5	2 oz.	10	0
Ham, boiled, lean	62	2 oz.	124	0
Heart	27	3 oz.	81	0
Kidneys, stewed	45	3 oz.	135	0
Lamb, roast leg	83	3 oz.	249	0
chop, grilled	108	3 oz.	324	0
roast shoulder	100	3 oz.	300	0
Liver, (ox), fried	81	4 oz.	342	0
Mutton, roast	83	3 oz.	249	0
Pork, medium fat leg, roast	90	3 oz.	270	0
cutlets, fried	155	3 oz.	465	0
chops, grilled, lean	92	3 oz.	276	0
Sausages, beef, fried	81	3 oz.	243	3
black	81	2 oz.	162	2
breakfast	82	2 oz.	164	2
pork, fried	93	4 oz.	372	3

Turkey, roast	56	2 oz.	112	0
Veal, roast	66	3 oz.	198	0

Sea Food

Cod, steamed	23	8 oz.	184	0
fried	58	8 oz.	464	0
Crab meat	36	3 oz.	108	0
Eel, stewed	106	3 oz.	318	0
Fish fingers	65 (each)	4 (3 oz.)	200	1
Fish paste	49	¾ oz.	36	0
Haddock, steamed	28	6 oz.	168	0
Herring, in vinegar	54	6 oz.	324	0
Lobster	34	3 oz.	102	0
Mackerel, boiled	39	6 oz.	234	0
Oysters, raw	14	(12) 4 oz.	56	0
Prawns, boiled	30	4 oz.	120	0
Salmon, red, fresh, steamed	57	4 oz.	216	0
canned	39	3 oz.	117	0
Sardines, solids + oils	84	2 oz.	168	0
solids, only	60	2 oz.	120	0
Shrimps, boiled	32	4 oz.	128	0
Sole, steamed	24	4 oz.	96	0

Miscellaneous

Beverages, orange, lemon, grapefruit squashes, various	36-39	2 oz.	72-78	4
Low calorie squash	3	2 oz.	6	0

Product	Calories per oz.	Average portion	Calories per portion	Carbo-hydrate units
Blancmange	34	6 oz.	210	0
Cocoa powder	128	½ oz.	64	0
Coffee	1	6 oz.	6	0
Doughnuts	101	(1) 4 oz.	404	12
Jam Roll	115	3 oz.	345	9
Mince pie	111	(1) 2 oz.	222	5
Sausage Roll	142	(1) 2 oz.	284	4
Soups, clear	5	8 oz.	40	0
Tea	1	6 oz.	6	0

Alcoholic Drinks

Product	Calories per oz.	Average portion	Calories per portion	Carbo-hydrate units *
Beer, 1 pint	8-11	1 pt.	160-220	4	8
Champagne	21	3 oz.	63	0	3
Ciders	11	10 oz.	110	2	6
Port	43	2 oz.	86	1	4.5
Sherry, dry	33	2 oz.	66	0	3
sweet	38	2 oz.	76	1	4
Spirits	63	1 oz.	63	0	3
Stout	10	10 oz.	100	0	5
Wines, white	21-26	4 oz.	84-102	0	4-5
red	18-20	4 oz.	72-80	0	3.5

* Including the carbohydrate equivalent of the alcoholic content.

Appendix C

Foods Grouped According to Calorie Values

These values are taken from "The Composition of Foods" by
R.A. McCance and E.M. Widdowson. H.M.S.O. London, 1967.
Medical Research Council. S.R.S. 297.

In the following groups of foods the calorie content of fruits and vegetables are calculated for fresh foodstuffs or those canned without syrup. The calorie content of fruits are increased considerably when stewed with sugar or canned in syrup.

	Meat	Fish	Fruit	Vegetables	Other
Very low in calories (0-5 calories per ounce)			Grapefruit Lemons Loganberries Rhubarb	Artichokes Asparagus Beans (French) Broccoli Brussell Sprouts Cabbage (cooked) Cauliflower (cooked) Egg Plant Marrow Mushrooms Onions Salad vegetables Turnips	Black coffee Lemon juice Low calorie drinks Bouillon Clear Soup Tea Tomato juice
Low in calories (5-15 calories per ounce)			Apples Apricots Blackberries	Beetroot Broad beans Carrots	Beer Cider

	Meat	Fish	Fruit	Vegetables	Other
Fairly low in calories (15-30 calories per ounce)	Brain Heart Tripe	Cod Haddock Oysters Prawns Sole	Cherries Gooseberries Melons Oranges Peaches Pears Pineapple Plums Raspberries Strawberries	Leeks Cabbage (raw) Cauliflower (raw) Spinach	without sugar or milk Jellies made with low calorie squash and gelatine Malted milk made without milk Milk (skimmed) Ovaltine made without milk Stout Yoghurt
Average calorific value (30-70 calories per ounce)	Chicken Goose Ham (lean) Kidneys Rabbit Turkey Veal	Herring Kippers Lobster Mackerel Pilchards Salmon	Avocadoes Bananas Grapes Figs Prunes	Baked Beans Corn (sweet) Olives Parsnips Peas Potatoes	Cottage cheese Champagne Jellies Milk Wines
				Potatoes (roast)	Blancmange Cream (thin) Dumplings Eggs Fruit gums Ice cream Macaroni

	Meat	Fish	Fruit	Vegetables	Other
High calorific value (70-120 calories per ounce)	Bacon Beef Duck Ham (lean and fat) Lamb Liver Mutton Sausages	Eels Sardines	Dates Raisins Sultanas	Potatoes (chipped)	Milk (evaporated) Milk puddings Port Sherry Spirits Squashes (neat) Yorkshire pudding Bread Breakfast cereals Cheese (Camembert, Edam, Danish Blue) Cheese spread Jam Milk (sweetened condensed) Sponge cake Sugar, sweets Suet puddings Syrup

Foods of Very High Calorific Value
(over 120 calories per ounce)

GROUP A. These products are very satisfying and can be taken in moderation provided they are not taken in conjunction with sugar or starch.

Butter, cooking fat, margarine. Olive oil, peanut butter, thick cream. Cheddar, Parmesan and Stilton cheese, cream cheese. Fatty Ham, Pork. Nuts.

GROUP B. These products are mainly sweet and tend to create an artificial appetite. They should be avoided at all costs, although some types contain less than 120 calories per ounce.

Biscuits, Doughnuts, Cake, Pastry, Shortbread, Cocoa powder, Chocolate.